Inflammatory Dermatoses: The Basics

Inflammatory Dermatoses: The Basics

Bruce R. Smoller, MD

Chair of Pathology
Professor of Pathology and Dermatology
University of Arkansas for Medical Sciences
Little Rock, Arkansas, USA

and

616,51
S666

Kim M. Hiatt, MD

Director of Dermatopathology
Associate Professor of Pathology and Dermatology
University of Arkansas for Medical Sciences
Little Rock, Arkansas, USA

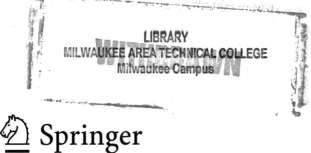

Springer

Bruce R. Smoller
Department of Pathology
University of Arkansas
 for Medical Sciences
4301 W. Markham Street
Little Rock, Arkansas 72205
USA
smollerbrucer@uams.edu

Kim M. Hiatt
Department of Pathology
University of Arkansas
 for Medical Sciences
4301 W. Markham Street
Little Rock, Arkansas 72205
USA
hiattkimm@uams.edu

ISBN 978-1-4419-6003-0   e-ISBN 978-1-4419-6004-7
DOI 10.1007/978-1-4419-6004-7
Springer New York Dordrecht Heidelberg London

Library of Congress Control Number: 2010926591

Printed on acid-free paper

Springer is part of Springer Science+Business Media (www.springer.com)

Preface

This volume is dedicated to inflammatory dermatoses. The intent of this volume is to provide a framework from which to classify this category of dermopathies. We have sought to include neither all variations of an entity nor subtleties of histologic features.

For each entity, a concise clinical presentation is given and the major histologic findings described are accompanied by quality photographs to illustrate these points. The most common dermatologic diseases and the most common histologic findings are presented. The meaning is to supplement the larger resources already available to the trainee. Our hope is that this bullet-point outline provides a meaning scaffold from which the reader can build as knowledge is acquired.

Contents

Acknowledgments

The images in this volume could not be made available without the efforts put forth by our dermatopathology laboratory staff. We work with an outstanding group dedicated to providing quality patient care. It is with their commitment to perfection that these images are possible. This volume is dedicated to the pioneer in this group Vicky Givens, who started the dermatopathology laboratory at University of Arkansas for Medical Sciences. She devoted her days to patient care through the pride she had in a perfectly cut specimen. Vicky lost her battle with breast cancer in 2009. She is missed, but the lab continues with the spirit of dedication that she instituted from her first adventure with this lab in 1997.

As always, Bruce Smoller wishes to acknowledge his wife, Laura, and two children, Jason and Gabriel, for their constant enthusiastic support and love. And, Dr. Hiatt would like to thank her husband, Jim, for his support and for the enthusiasm of her children, Stephanie, Nicholas, Kaitlyn, and Natalie, who have as much fun saying "dermatopathology" as she does teaching it.

Chapter 1
Superficial Perivascular Dermatitis

- Superficial perivascular dermatitis

  - Inflammatory dermatoses involving venules in superficial vascular plexus
  - Other histologic changes help with further classification

- Superficial perivascular dermatitis (SPD)

  - Without epidermal changes

    o Lymphocytic infiltrate
    o Mixed infiltrate

  - With epidermal changes

    o Interface/vacuolar and lichenoid dermatitis (Chapter 2)
    o Spongiotic dermatitis (Chapter 3)
    o Psoriasiform dermatitis (Chapter 4, Table 1.1)

Table 1.1 Superficial perivascular lymphohistiocytic dermatitis without epidermal changes

Pigmented purpuric eruption
Viral exanthem
Gyrate erythema
Dermatophytoses
Post-inflammatory pigment alteration
Rocky mountain spotted fever
Polymorphous light eruption

B.R. Smoller, K.M. Hiatt, *Inflammatory Dermatoses: The Basics*,
DOI 10.1007/978-1-4419-6004-7_1,
© Springer Science+Business Media, LLC 2010

- Pigmented purpuric eruption, Schamberg variant (progressive pigmentary dermatosis)

  - Clinical

    o Erythematous, non-blanching patches
    o Usually on lower extremities, pre-tibial
    o Most common in middle-aged men
    o May be related to drug exposure in some cases
    o Controversial relationship with mycosis fungoides

      Recent literature suggests possibility of progression

    o Multiple subtypes of pigmented purpuric eruption

      This is the most common; all other subtypes demonstrate epidermal changes

  - Histologic findings

    o Superficial perivascular lymphohistiocytic infiltrate
    o Eosinophils not common
    o Mild spongiosis and exocytosis
    o Hemorrhage and hemosiderin surrounding vessels in superficial vascular plexus
    o Perl's iron or Prussian blue stain often helpful in demonstrating dermal hemosiderin deposition (necessary to document chronicity of process) (Figs. 1.1 and 1.2)

- Viral exanthem

  - Clinical

    o Morbilliform (measles-like) eruption
    o Erythematous papules and macules – usually rapid onset
    o Resolves rapidly without sequelae in most cases

  - Histologic findings

    o Superficial perivascular lymphohistiocytic infiltrate
    o Inflammation does not usually extend into deeper dermis
    o Eosinophils very uncommon
    o Slight exocytosis, epidermal spongiosis, and basal vacuolopathy

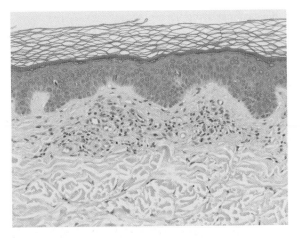

Fig. 1.1 Pigmented purpuric eruption, Schamberg variant, shows a mild superficial perivascular lymphohistiocytic infiltrate. Erythrocyte extravasation is present. The overlying epidermis is uninvolved

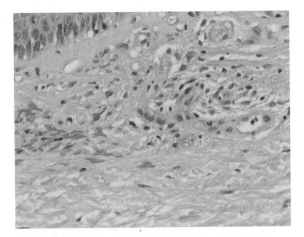

Fig. 1.2 Pigmented purpuric eruption, Schamberg variant. This high-power image shows perivascular erythrocyte extravasation. Hemosiderosis is variable, depending on the duration of disease, and can be nearly non-existent as in this case

- ○ Occasional dying keratinocytes, but very few
- ○ *Non-specific findings – hard to establish diagnosis without clinical correlation* (Figs. 1.3 and 1.4)

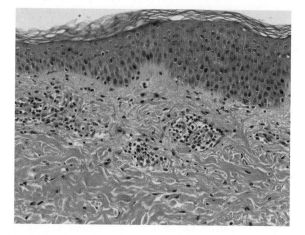

Fig. 1.3 This viral exanthem shows a superficial perivascular lymphohistiocytic infiltrate with no alterations in the overlying epidermis

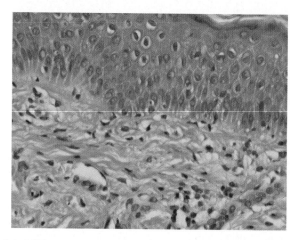

Fig. 1.4 Mild spongiosis and interface degeneration are seen in this viral exanthem

- Gyrate erythema

    - Clinical

        o Most commonly refers to erythema annulare centrifugum, but also includes erythema gyratum repens, erythema chronicum migrans, other less common eruptions
        o Annular, erythematous lesions on trunk
        o Slow outward extension of plaques in some cases
        o Peripheral, delicate scale

    - Histologic findings

        o Almost entirely lymphoid infiltrate in a perivascular distribution
        o Eosinophils may rarely present in small numbers
        o "Tight cuffing" of lymphocytes around vessels of the superficial vascular plexus
        o Some cases also involve deeper vascular plexus
        o Scant parakeratotic scale with mild underlying spongiosis if peripheral scale is biopsied
        o Plasma cells present in small numbers in erythema chronicum migrans, but not usually in erythema annulare centrifugum (Figs. 1.5, 1.6, and 1.7)

- Dermatophytosis

    - Clinical

        o Tinea versicolor, caused by *Pityrosporum versicolor*, classically shows minimal epidermal change
        o *Trichophyton*, *Epidermophyton*, and *Microsporum* species cause dermatophytoses that are classically more inflammatory with epidermal changes, but may be missed with a low clinical threshold
        o Scaly, erythematous to red-brown annular lesions
        o Can occur anywhere on body (head and neck less common in adults)
        o Often very pruritic

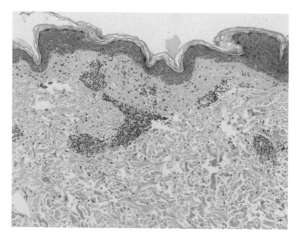

Fig. 1.5 Erythema annulare centrifugum is characterized by a lympho-histiocytic infiltrate tightly cuffed around the vessels

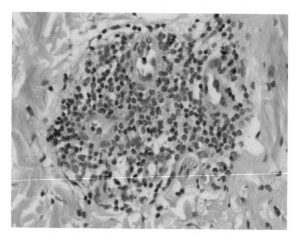

Fig. 1.6 Erythema annulare centrifugum characteristically has a lympho-histiocytic infiltrate. Plasma cells may be seen; neutrophils and eosinophils are not characteristic

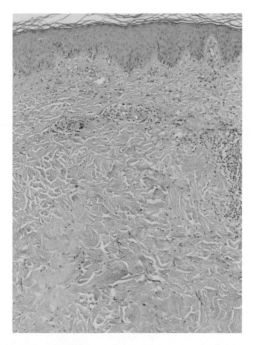

Fig. 1.7 Erythema chronicum migrans shows a superficial perivascular lymphohistiocytic infiltrate without significant epidermal involvement

- Histologic findings

  o Small foci of parakeratotic keratin
  o Minimal superficial perivascular inflammation (occasionally eosinophils or neutrophils may be present)
  o Mild spongiosis
  o PASD stains often helpful in making diagnosis – neutrophils in the stratum corneum may be a hint to requesting a PASD stain (Figs. 1.8, 1.9, 1.10, and 1.11)

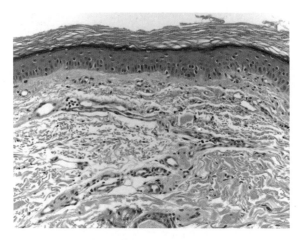

Fig. 1.8 Tinea versicolor, caused by *Pityrosporum versicolor*, has a very mild superficial perivascular lymphocytic infiltrate. Parakeratosis in this example is florid, but may be very mild and focal

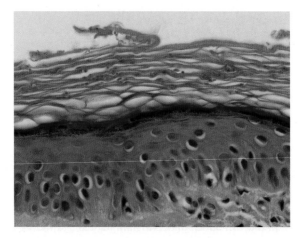

Fig. 1.9 On close inspection of the stratum corneum, hypae and yeast forms may be seen without the assistance of special stains, such as PAS

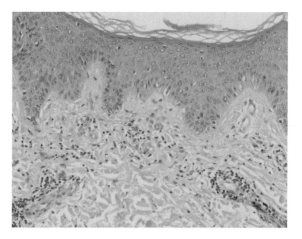

Fig. 1.10 Dermatophytoses may show only superficial perivascular lymphocytic infiltrate. Focal hyperkeratosis or parakeratosis may be the only clue to the dermatophyte

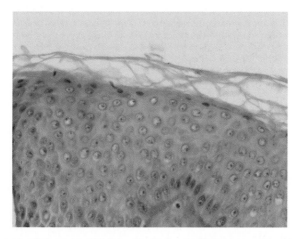

Fig. 1.11 PAS staining highlights the hyphae in the stratum corneum in this minimally inflamed dermatophyte infection

- Post-inflammatory pigment alteration

  - Clinical

    - ○ Areas of mottled hyper- or hypopigmentation
    - ○ It is difficult, if not impossible, to distinguish based on histologic sections if the biopsy is from a hyper- or hypopigmented region (hence nomenclature)
    - ○ Often occurs following an inflammatory process with erythema (may be clinically undetected)

  - Histologic findings

    - ○ Variable lymphohistiocytic infiltrate around superficial vascular plexus
    - ○ Melanophages present in papillary dermis
    - ○ If still active, there are mild interface changes with basal vacuolization and dying keratinocytes
    - ○ Papillary dermal fibrosis is present if the process is chronic
    - ○ *Diagnosis is not specific, but rather engenders a differential diagnosis including most interface dermatoses as well as erythema dyschromicum perstans* (Figs. 1.12, 1.13, and 1.14)

- Rocky mountain spotted fever (RMSF)

  - Clinical

    - ○ Caused by tick transmission of *Rickettsia rickettsii*
    - ○ Non-blanching erythematous papules and macules
    - ○ Rapid dissemination
    - ○ Petechia starts on acral site and spreads to trunk
    - ○ Looks like leukocytoclastic vasculitis
    - ○ Patients have systemic symptoms and are acutely ill

  - Histologic findings

    - ○ True "lymphocytic vasculitis"; fibrinoid necrosis of the vascular wall may be seen
    - ○ Purely lymphoid infiltrate
    - ○ Endothelial cell swelling

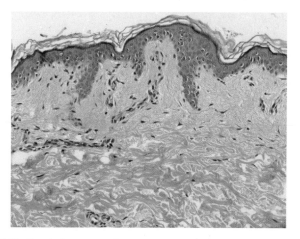

Fig. 1.12 Post-inflammatory pigment alteration shows a very mild superficial perivascular lymphohistiocytic infiltrate. Melanophages in the dermis may be very challenging to find on scanning power

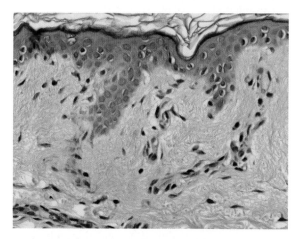

Fig. 1.13 Melanophages in post-inflammatory pigment alteration may be sparse and detected only by high-power investigation

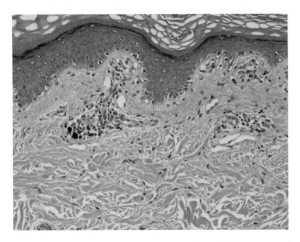

Fig. 1.14 In chronic cases, the melanophages of post-inflammatory pigment alteration are more pronounced

- o Erythrocyte extravasation
- o Thrombosed dermal blood vessels
- o Apparent vascular damage of vessels throughout dermis (superficial and deep vascular plexuses) (Figs. 1.15 and 1.16)

- Polymorphous light eruption (PMLE)

  - Clinical

    - o Papules, plaques, vesicles, and erythema (polymorphous lesions)
    - o Sun-exposed areas
    - o Recurs annually at time of first exposure to sun in the spring
    - o Body develops tolerance to UV light as summer progresses and disease diminishes and ultimately abates

  - Histologic findings

    - o Superficial perivascular lymphohistiocytic infiltrate in early lesions

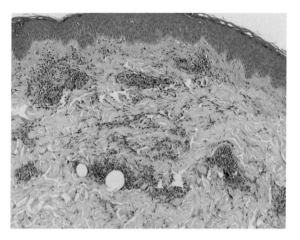

Fig. 1.15 Rocky mountain spotted fever, caused by *Rickettsia rickettsii*, shows a moderate perivascular lymphocytic infiltrate with endothelial swelling and erythrocyte extravasation

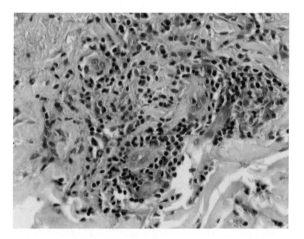

Fig. 1.16 Perivascular lymphocytic infiltrate, endothelial swelling, and erythrocyte extravasation are characteristic, but not specific, of rickettsial infections. Patchy fibrinoid necrosis of the involved vessels, not seen in this specimen, can occasionally be seen

- o Superficial and deep perivascular lymphohistiocytic infiltrate in established lesions
- o Slight spongiosis and exocytosis of lymphocytes may be present
- o Papillary dermal edema is marked in some cases
- o The inflammatory infiltrate may extend into the deep vascular plexus
- o Minimal eosinophils may be seen
- o Less common variant presents without papillary dermal edema and a deep lymphoid infiltrate
- o Histologic changes vary in concert with clinically polymorphous appearance (Figs. 1.17, 1.18, 1.19, and 1.20)

- SPD without epidermal changes

  - Mixed inflammatory infiltrate

    - o Urticaria
    - o Arthropod bite reaction
    - o Pruritic urticarial papules and plaques of pregnancy

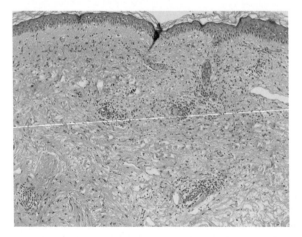

Fig. 1.17 Polymorphous light eruption shows a perivascular lymphocytic infiltrate involving the superficial vascular plexus as well as mid and deep dermal vessels in more evolved lesions

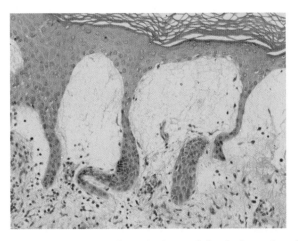

Fig. 1.18 Prominent papillary edema is characteristic of polymorphous light eruption

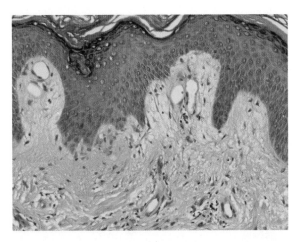

Fig. 1.19 In polymorphous light eruption, papillary dermal edema may be minimal to moderate, as in this case

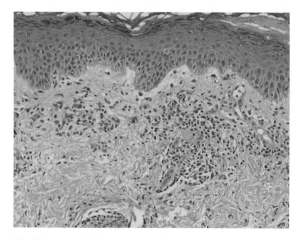

Fig. 1.20 This case of polymorphous light eruption further exemplifies the polymorphous nature of the infiltrate showing perivascular inflammation with spill-over into the interstitium and only minimal papillary dermal edema

- Urticaria
  - Clinical
    - Transient erythematous patches and plaques without epidermal changes
    - Dermal wheals (consisting of edema)
    - Lesions persist (by definition) less than 24 h
  - Histologic findings
    - May look like normal skin
    - Close inspection reveals slight perivascular edema (may not be perceptible)
    - Sparse infiltrate of lymphocytes, neutrophils, scattered eosinophils, and mast cells around superficial vascular plexus
    - No epidermal changes (Figs. 1.21 and 1.22)

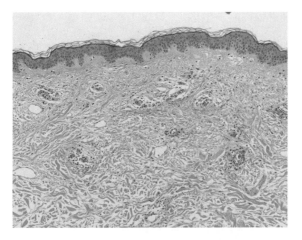

Fig. 1.21 Urticaria on low power, looks like normal skin

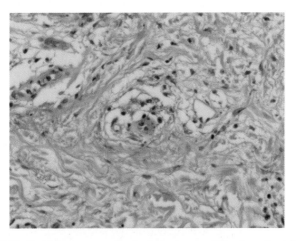

Fig. 1.22 On higher power, urticaria shows a very mild perivascular inflammatory infiltrate with lymphocytes and rare neutrophils or eosinophils. Perivascular edema can also be appreciated

- Arthropod bite reaction

  - Clinical

    - Multiple papules with central areas of epidermal disruption (puncta)
    - Surrounding erythema and swelling

  - Histologic findings

    - Punctum with parakeratosis and spongiosis (may be seen on sections)
    - Superficial (and deep) infiltrate of lymphocytes with abundant eosinophils
    - Interstitial eosinophils are seen characteristically
    - Neutrophils are variably present
    - May extend into subcutaneous fat
    - Dermal hemorrhage may be present
    - *Interstitial inflammation in addition to perivascular infiltrate may be diagnostic clue* (Figs. 1.23, 1.24, and 1.25)

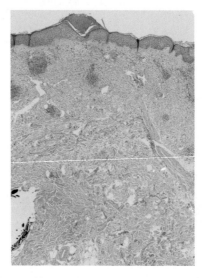

Fig. 1.23 Arthropod bite reactions show a variably intense inflammatory infiltrate around the vessels and extending into the interstitium. The epidermis, in this example, shows the punctum in the epidermis with focal parakeratosis with surrounding epidermal spongiosis

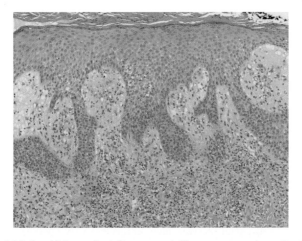

Fig. 1.24 In addition to the inflammatory infiltrate, some sections of arthropod bite reactions may show epidermal acanthosis, hypergranulosis, parakeratosis, and spongiosis, secondary to rubbing or excoriation

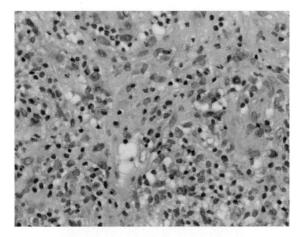

Fig. 1.25 On high power, the arthropod bite reaction shows numerous eosinophils in the inflammatory infiltrate

- Pruritic urticarial papules and plaques of pregnancy (PUPPP)

  - Clinical

    - Occurs in third trimester of pregnancy
    - Most common in first pregnancies, rarely recurs in subsequent ones
    - Peri-umbilical papules and plaques
    - Intensely pruritic
    - Not associated with any fetal problems
    - Usually biopsied to distinguish from pemphigoides (herpes) gestationis

  - Histologic findings

    - Superficial perivascular infiltrate of lymphocytes and eosinophils
    - Mild epidermal spongiosis and exocytosis

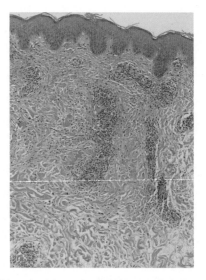

Fig. 1.26 Pruritic urticarial papules and plaques of pregnancy have a superficial perivascular lymphocytic infiltrate with increased eosinophils. The epidermis shows mild acanthosis, hypergranulosis, and hyperkeratosis secondary to excoriation

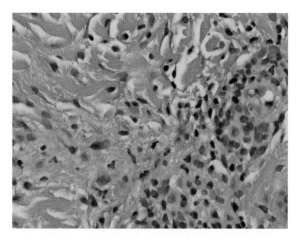

Fig. 1.27   Pruritic urticarial papules and plaques of pregnancy show increased eosinophils in the inflammatory infiltrate

- ○ *Difficult to distinguish (on histologic grounds) from mild contact dermatitis or photo-allergic drug eruption* (Figs. 1.26 and 1.27)

Chapter 2
Lichenoid/Vacuolar Dermatitis

- Superficial perivascular dermatitis (SPD) with epidermal changes
  - Vacuolar/interface changes
  - Lichenoid changes
- Interface dermatitis
  - Superficial perivascular lymphocytic infiltrate
  - Exocytosis of single lymphocytes into overlying epidermis
  - Basal vacuolization
  - Dying keratinocytes
  - Dermal–epidermal junction not obscured (Table 2.1)

Table 2.1 SPD with epidermal changes – vacuolar/interface changes

Erythema multiforme
Graft vs. host disease
Lupus erythematosus
Dermatomyositis
Lichen sclerosus
Radiodermatitis
Pityriasis lichenoides (chronica)
Fixed drug eruption

- Erythema multiforme
  - Clinical

B.R. Smoller, K.M. Hiatt, *Inflammatory Dermatoses: The Basics*,
DOI 10.1007/978-1-4419-6004-7_2,
© Springer Science+Business Media, LLC 2010

- o Targetoid lesions
- o Most common on acral sites
- o Associated with herpes simplex in most cases
- o Also associated with *Mycoplasma pneumoniae*, drug exposure
- o Minor variant not associated with severe sequelae
- o Two "major" forms of erythema multiforme (somewhat controversial in literature)

  Stevens–Johnson syndrome – blistering process involving mucosal surfaces, associated more intimately with drug exposure and less with infectious diseases than the minor form

  Toxic epidermal necrolysis – desquamation of large sheets of epidermis, associated almost exclusively with drug exposure; very high mortality rate

- – Histologic

  - o Orthokeratotic keratin
  - o Superficial perivascular lymphohistiocytic infiltrate with scattered eosinophils
  - o Exocytosis of lymphocytes into epidermis
  - o Lymphocytic infiltrate usually relatively slight
  - o Basal vacuolization
  - o Necrotic keratinocytes at all levels of epidermis
  - o *Accentuation of dying keratinocytes in acrosyringia may be hint of drug-induced eruption*
  - o Stevens–Johnson syndrome demonstrates identical histologic changes occurring on mucosal surfaces
  - o Toxic epidermal necrolysis is characterized by:

    full-thickness epidermal necrosis
    subepidermal blister formation
    relatively slight lymphocytic infiltrate

    (Figs. 2.1, 2.2, 2.3, and 2.4)

- • Graft vs. host disease

  - – Clinical

    - o Acute and chronic forms associated with varying times post-transplantation

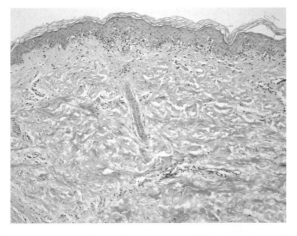

Fig. 2.1 Erythema multiforme demonstrates a mild interface dermatitis with minimal inflammatory infiltrate in the deeper dermis. Original magnification 100×

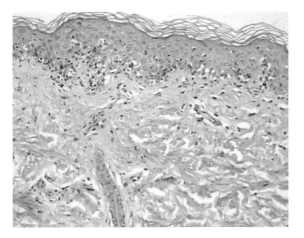

Fig. 2.2 At higher magnification, abundant dying keratinocytes, basal vacuolization, and infiltration of the epidermis by lymphocytes are apparent in erythema multiforme. Original magnification 200×

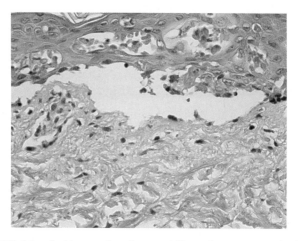

Fig. 2.3 More florid cases of erythema multiforme demonstrate a subepidermal blister caused by necrosis of keratinocytes. Original magnification 400×

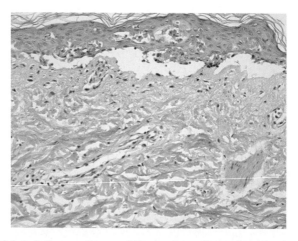

Fig. 2.4 In bullous erythema multiforme, sheets of necrotic epidermis separate from the underlying dermis. The changes are similar in toxic epidermal necrolysis, but the epidermis demonstrates more complete necrolysis and there is a relatively scant lymphocytic infiltrate. Original magnification 200×

- o Difficult to diagnose prior to 3 weeks following transplantation
- o Must be distinguished from eruption of cutaneous lymphocyte recovery
- o Maculopapular eruption – commonly involves ears and palms
- o Often associated with gastrointestinal symptoms and oral lesions

- – Histologic

  - o Superficial perivascular lymphocytic infiltrate – sparse
  - o Eosinophils quite uncommon
  - o Exocytosis into epidermis with dying keratinocytes – majority in basal layer
  - o Melanophages in chronic forms (also lichenoid and sclerodermatous changes)
  - o *Difficult to distinguish from erythema multiforme without history* (Figs. 2.5, 2.6, 2.7, 2.8, 2.9, and 2.10)

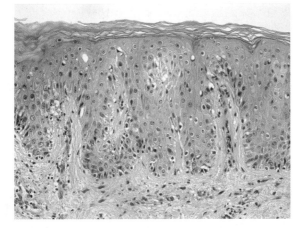

Fig. 2.5 Grade I graft vs. host disease (GVHD) is characterized by a mild spongiosis with slight basal vacuolization. The changes are not specific. Original magnification 200×

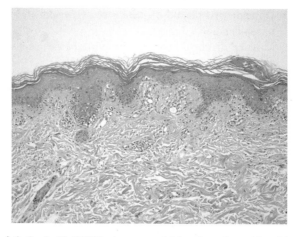

Fig. 2.6 Grade II GVHD shows a mild interface dermatitis with scattered dermal lymphocytes and basal vacuolization at low power. Original magnification 100×

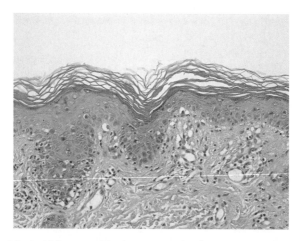

Fig. 2.7 At higher magnification, scattered dying keratinocytes are seen surrounded by intraepidermal lymphocytes in grade II GVHD. Original magnification 200×

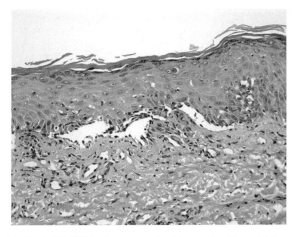

Fig. 2.8 Grade III GVHD is characterized by a subepidermal blister with dying keratinocytes and a mild lymphocytic infiltrate. Original magnification 200×

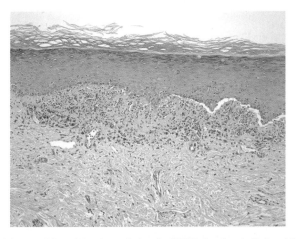

Fig. 2.9 The lichenoid variant of chronic GVHD is often indistinguishable histologically from lichen planus and requires clinical correlation. There is a band-like infiltrate of lymphocytes, a subepidermal separation, and an acanthotic epidermis, often with hypergranulosis. Original magnification 100×

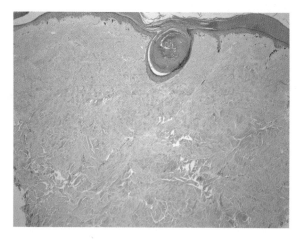

Fig. 2.10 Sclerodermatoid chronic GVHD is quite similar to scleroderma with loss of appendages, dermal sclerosis, and a minimal inflammatory infiltrate. There is often pigment incontinence, evidence of an antecedent interface dermatitis. Original magnification 40×

- Lupus erythematosus (LE)

  - Clinical

    o Discoid lesions

      Annular, erythematous patches with overlying thick scale
      Follicular plugging clinically apparent
      Most common on sun-exposed sites

    o Systemic LE with less pronounced changes and may occur in sun-protected areas
    o Subacute cutaneous LE – more pronounced histologic changes (but too much overlap to make distinction based upon histologic changes)

  - Histologic

    o Superficial (and deep) perivascular and peri-appendageal infiltrate of lymphocytes and rare plasma cells
    o Epidermal atrophy

- o Basal vacuolization
- o Rare dying keratinocytes (more extensive in subacute cutaneous LE)
- o Follicular plugging
- o Dermal mucin (slight) (Figs. 2.11, 2.12, 2.13, and 2.14)

- Dermatomyositis

  - Clinical

    - o Heliotrope erythema around eyes
    - o Gottron's papules on dorsal fingers
    - o Erythematous patches with poikilodermatous mottling on chest and back

  - Histologic

    - o Mild superficial perivascular infiltrate of lymphocytes
    - o No peri-appendageal or deep component to infiltrate
    - o Basal vacuolization, epidermal atrophy

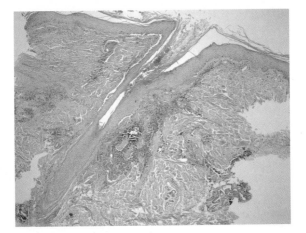

Fig. 2.11 Lupus erythematosus (LE) is characterized by a superficial and deep lymphocytic infiltrate with interface changes and peri-appendageal inflammation. Original magnification 40×

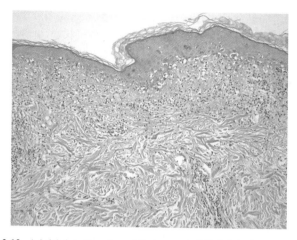

Fig. 2.12 A brisk interface dermatitis is seen in LE. Original magnification 100×

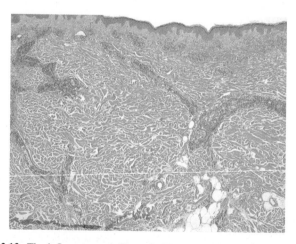

Fig. 2.13 The inflammatory infiltrate in LE extends deeply into the dermis and surrounds blood vessels as well as dermal appendages. Original magnification 40×

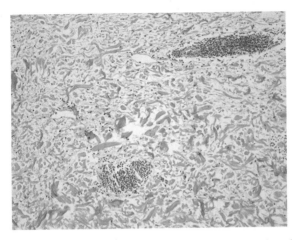

Fig. 2.14 A colloidal iron stain (pH 4.5) demonstrates abundant dermal mucin in most cases of LE. Original magnification 100×

- o Pigment incontinence with melanophages in dermis
- o Abundant dermal mucin (especially in Gottron's papules)
- o *Resembles mild lupus erythematosus with abundant mucin* (Figs. 2.15 and 2.16)

- Lichen sclerosus

  - Clinical

    - o Porcelain white lesions with tissue paper-like hyperker-atosis
    - o Apparent epidermal atrophy
    - o Usually peri-genital, but can be seen extra-genitally
    - o Similar changes associated with some cases of morphea
    - o Some association between genital LS and squamous cell carcinoma (weak)

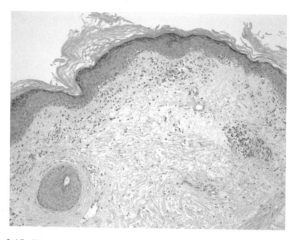

Fig. 2.15 Dermatomyositis demonstrates a relatively slight interface dermatitis with a superficial perivascular lymphocytic infiltrate. Peri-appendageal inflammation is not prominent. Original magnification 100×

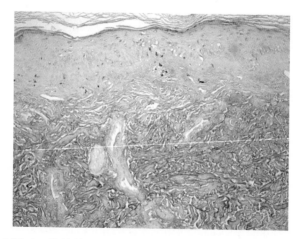

Fig. 2.16 A colloidal iron stain (pH 4.5) demonstrates abundant mucin in the superficial dermis in dermatomyositis. Original magnification 100×

- Histologic

  o Early lesions – dense band-like infiltrate of lymphocytes (more "lichenoid" than "interface pattern – see below)
  o Well-developed lesions

    Papillary dermal expansion and homogenization
    Mild superficial perivascular lymphoid infiltrate with exocytosis
    Basal vacuolization
    Follicular plugging

  o Late-stage lesions – epidermal atrophy, minimal inflammation, pigmentary incontinence with melanophages
  o *May resemble lupus erythematosus, but dermal homogenization helps to distinguish as does lack of deep or periappendageal inflammation in lichen sclerosis* (Figs. 2.17 and 2.18)

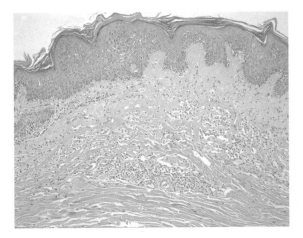

Fig. 2.17 Early lichen sclerosis (LS) demonstrates a perivascular to band-like infiltrate of lymphocytes that may be separated from the dermal–epidermal junction by variable amounts of homogenized eosinophilic material. The epidermis is not atrophic. Original magnification 100×

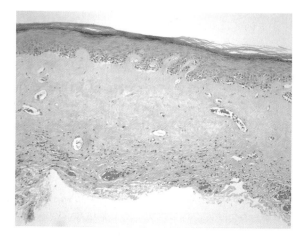

Fig. 2.18 Well-developed lesions of LS demonstrate marked epidermal atrophy with overlying orthokeratotic hyperkeratosis and markedly thickened and homogenized papillary dermis. Any lymphocytic infiltrate is relatively sparse. Original magnification 100×

- Radiation dermatitis

  - Clinical

    - Epidermal atrophy
    - Telangiectasia
    - Mottled hypo- and hyperpigmentation
    - Dermal sclerosis in long-standing, extensive lesions

  - Histologic

    - Superficial perivascular lymphoid infiltrate – sparse
    - Homogenization of papillary dermis
    - Melanophages underlying basal vacuolization
    - Radiation fibroblasts
    - Thick-walled blood vessels with endothelial cell swelling
    - "Radiation fibroblasts" between collagen bundles – cytologically atypical – enlarged, hyperchromatic nuclei (Figs. 2.19 and 2.20)

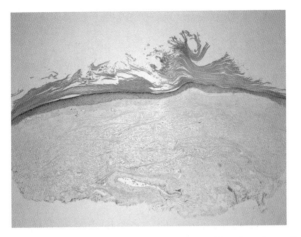

Fig. 2.19 In radiation dermatitis, there is a thinned epidermis and a markedly sclerotic dermis that may demonstrate a slight perivascular lymphocytic infiltrate. Early lesions (not shown here) may demonstrate features of a mild interface dermatitis. Original magnification 40×

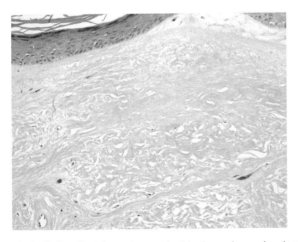

Fig. 2.20 Radiation fibroblasts, characterized by hyperchromasia, pleomorphism, and florid cytologic atypia, are seen coursing through the sclerotic dermis. Original magnification 200×

- Pityriasis lichenoides (chronica) (PLC)

  - Clinical

    - Multiple papules on trunk and extremities with overlying scale
    - Ulceration not frequent
    - Often in adolescents/young adults
    - Papules at all stages of development concurrently
    - Relatively asymptomatic

  - Histologic

    - Superficial perivascular lymphoid infiltrate with exocytosis
    - Basal vacuolization and rare dying keratinocytes
    - Eosinophils rare
    - Overlying parakeratosis
    - Scant dermal and epidermal hemorrhage
    - *Parakeratosis helps distinguish from erythema multiforme* (Figs. 2.21 and 2.22)

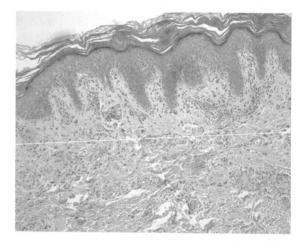

Fig. 2.21 Pityriasis lichenoides chronica (PLC) demonstrates confluent parakeratosis, exocytosis of lymphocytes into the epidermis, and a mild superficial perivascular lymphocytic infiltrate in the dermis. Original magnification 100×

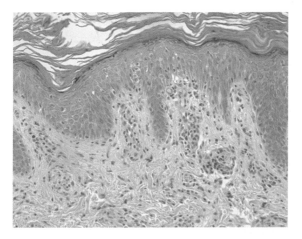

Fig. 2.22 In PLC, scattered dying keratinocytes may be seen and slight papillary dermal hemorrhage is often found near the lymphocytic infiltrate. Original magnification 200×

- Fixed drug eruption

  - Clinical

    o Circular erythematous eruption appears abruptly after ingestion of offending agent
    o Often singular on first occurrence and multiple with subsequent recurrences
    o May become bullous when severe
    o Heals with post-inflammatory hyperpigmentation
    o Occurs on face, genitals, buttocks most commonly
    o Associated with many medications

  - Histologic

    o Interface dermatitis with dying keratinocytes within and above basal layer
    o Eosinophils often present
    o Early lesions may have neutrophils
    o Pigment incontinence usually found, especially in recurrent lesions

  ○ *Inflammation usually extends deeper in dermis than in erythema multiforme* (Figs. 2.23 and 2.24)

● Lichenoid dermatitis

  – Band-like infiltrate of lymphocytes along the dermal–epidermal junction
  – Exocytosis of lymphocytes into epidermis
  – Dying keratinocytes, most apparent in lower layers of epidermis
  – Basal vacuolization
  – Infiltrate and keratinocyte damage so intense that dermal–epidermal junction focally obscured (Table 2.2)

● Lichen planus

  – Clinical

    ○ Pruritic, polygonal, purple papules on ventral surfaces of wrists
    ○ Also can be in any other body site

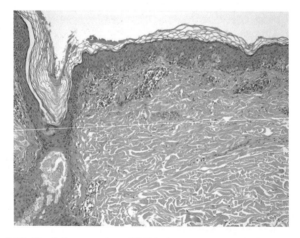

Fig. 2.23 Fixed drug eruptions (FDEs) demonstrate an interface dermatitis with multiple dying keratinocytes within and above the basal layer. Original magnification 100×

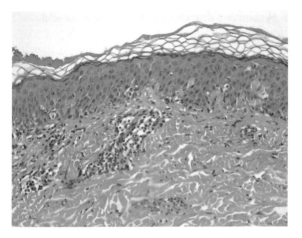

Fig. 2.24 In most biopsies of FDE, there is pronounced pigment incontinence in the papillary dermis. Original magnification 200×

Table 2.2   SPD with epidermal changes – lichenoid changes

Lichen planus
Lichenoid drug eruption
Lichenoid keratosis
Pityriasis lichenoides chronica (see above)
Mycosis fungoides (see Volume IV)
Pigmented purpuric eruption
Lichen striatus
Lichen nitidus
Secondary syphilis

- o Overlying hyperkeratosis (linear) – Wickham's striae
- o Oral lichen planus ulcerates – associated with squamous cell carcinoma in long-standing lesions

- – Histologic

    - o Epidermal hyperplasia
    - o Hyperkeratosis, but not parakeratosis
    - o Wedge-shaped hypergranulosis centered around acrosyringia

- o Band-like lymphoid infiltrate focally obscures dermal–epidermal junction
- o Lymphoid infiltrate does not extend deeper into dermis
- o Dying keratinocytes (colloid/Civatte bodies)
- o Eosinophils most unusual (Figs. 2.25, 2.26, and 2.27)

- • Lichenoid drug eruption

  - – Clinical

    - o Lesions resemble lichen planus
    - o Often can be associated temporarily with initiation of new medication (long list of implicated drugs)

  - – Histologic

    - o *Differs from LP by potential presence of eosinophils, deeper infiltrate, and parakeratosis*
    - o *None of these features are invariably present, so may be impossible to distinguish without clinical history* (Figs. 2.28 and 2.29)

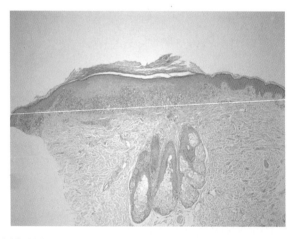

Fig. 2.25 Lichen planus is characterized by a flat-topped papule with overlying orthokeratotic hyperkeratosis. Original magnification 40×

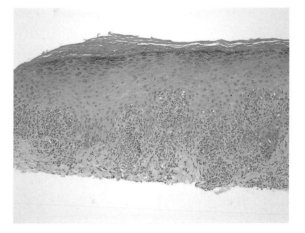

Fig. 2.26 In LP, there is a brisk lichenoid infiltrate of lymphocytes that obscures the dermal–epidermal junction. There is a wedge-shaped hypergranulosis and an acanthotic epidermis with saw-toothed rete ridges. Original magnification 100×

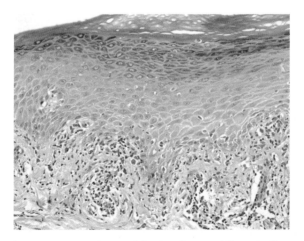

Fig. 2.27 LP is characterized by dying keratinocytes (Civatte bodies, cytoid bodies) and often demonstrates pigment incontinence, evidence of keratinocyte destruction by the dense infiltrate of lymphocytes at the dermal–epidermal junction. Original magnification 200×

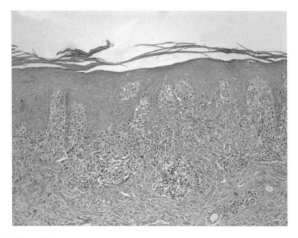

Fig. 2.28 A lichenoid drug eruption may be histologically indistinguishable from lichen planus. Occasional plasma cells or eosinophils (not seen in this case) may be a hint as to a drug-induced etiology for the eruption. Original magnification 100×

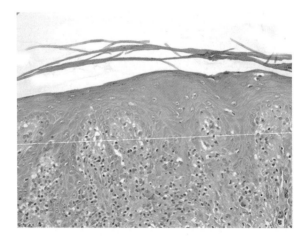

Fig. 2.29 Lichenoid drug eruptions may demonstrate overlying parakeratosis, a feature not usually found in lichen planus. Original magnification 200×

- Lichenoid keratosis

  - Clinical

    o Chest, back, upper extremities
    o Middle-aged to elderly patients
    o Scaly, slightly erythematous papule or plaque
    o May be slightly hyperpigmented
    o Clinical differential diagnosis includes basal cell carcinoma, seborrheic keratosis

  - Histologic

    o May be histologically indistinguishable from LP
    o Also may demonstrate

      Parakeratosis
      Eosinophils
      Deeper infiltrate of lymphocytes than in LP
      Less pronounced obstruction of dermal–epidermal junction (Fig. 2.30)

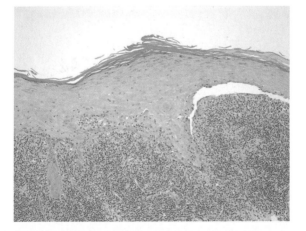

Fig. 2.30 While parakeratosis and eosinophils may be seen in some lichenoid keratoses, in many cases, biopsies from these lesions are indistinguishable from lichen planus. Clinical history is the best discriminator in these cases. Original magnification 200×

- Lichen striatus

  - Clinical

    ○ Most common in children and teenagers
    ○ Erythematous papules in a linear distribution
    ○ Scale on surface

  - Histologic

    ○ Superficial (and deep) perivascular and peri-appendageal (especially peri-eccrine) infiltrate
    ○ Band-like infiltrate at dermal–epidermal junction – does not usually totally obscure
    ○ *Resembles lupus erythematosus, but no mucin, different clinical presentation* (Figs. 2.31, 2.32, and 2.33)

- Lichen nitidus

  - Clinical

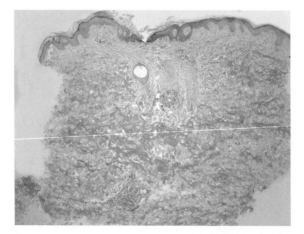

Fig. 2.31 Lichen striatus demonstrates interface dermatitis and deep, dense peri-eccrine inflammation similar to the changes seen in lupus erythematosus. However, unlike in lupus erythematosus, there is no epidermal atrophy, follicular plugging, or mucin deposition. Original magnification 40×

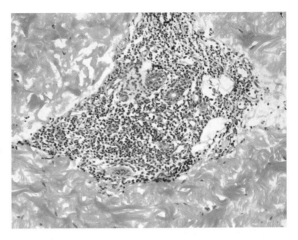

Fig. 2.32 A deep infiltrate of lymphocytes is present around eccrine structures in lichen striatus. Original magnification 200×

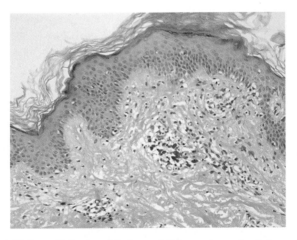

Fig. 2.33 In well-developed lesions of lichen striatus, the inflammatory infiltrate may be less intense, leaving only pigment incontinence in the papillary dermis, evidence of an antecedent interface dermatitis with dying keratinocytes. Original magnification 200×

- o Tiny flesh-colored papules (usually about 1 mm in diameter)
- o Usually asymptomatic to minimally pruritic
- o Often on penis, forearms
- o Rarely occurs in conjunction with lichen planus

- Histologic features

- o "Ball-and-claw" appearance
- o Epidermal hyperplasia with elongated rete ridges
- o Focal parakeratosis (only over area with dermal inflammatory infiltrate)
- o Lymphohistiocytic infiltrate along dermal–epidermal junction with some exocytosis
- o Occasional multinucleated cells
- o No eosinophils or plasma cells (Figs. 2.34 and 2.35)

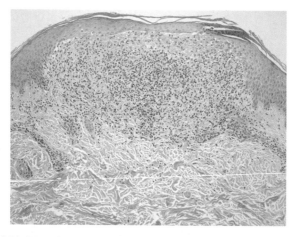

Fig. 2.34 Lichen nitidus is characterized by a "ball-and-claw" type of inflammatory infiltrate with a small aggregate of lymphocytes and histiocytes pushed up against the epidermis, with elongated rete ridges surrounding the infiltrate. There is often overlying parakeratosis. Original magnification 100×

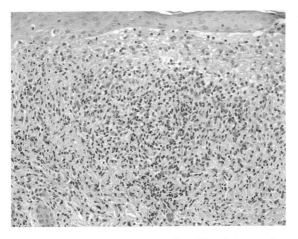

Fig. 2.35 The infiltrate in lichen nitidus consists of lymphocytes and scattered histiocytes. Original magnification 200×

- Secondary syphilis

  - Clinical features

    o "Great imitator" – can mimic many other dermatoses
    o Often resembles pityriasis rosea

      Erythematous annular patches
      Delicate peripheral scale

    o Lesions frequently on palms and soles – helps to differentiate from many other dermatoses that characteristically spare acral sites
    o Patchy "moth-eaten" alopecia may be present
    o Lesions almost never ulcerate

  - Histologic features

    o Variable parakeratosis
    o Frequently psoriasiform epidermal hyperplasia

- ○ Lichenoid (or more frequently, band-like, i.e., not obscuring the dermal–epidermal junction) infiltrate of lymphocytes
- ○ Plasma cells present as a minority population within inflammatory infiltrate
- ○ Frequent extension of infiltrate into deeper dermis
- ○ Organisms difficult to find using Warthin–Starry stain
- ○ Monoclonal anti-spirochetal antibodies are more sensitive in detecting organisms, usually along dermal–epidermal junction or near endothelial cells in superficial vascular plexus
- ○ *Constellation of psoriasiform epidermal hyperplasia, band-like infiltrate of lymphocytes, and extension of infiltrate into the deeper dermis raise limited differential diagnosis*

  Secondary syphilis
  Mycosis fungoides
  Lichen striatus

  (Figs. 2.36, 2.37, 2.38, and 2.39)

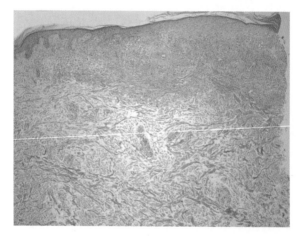

Fig. 2.36 Secondary syphilis demonstrates a band-like inflammatory infiltrate along with a superficial and deep perivascular infiltrate. There may be psoriasiform elongation of the rete ridges. Original magnification 40×

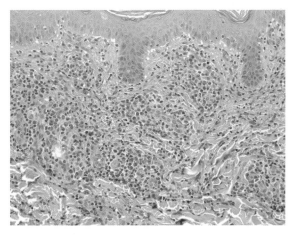

Fig. 2.37 The inflammatory infiltrate in secondary syphilis consists of lymphocytes admixed with plasma cells. Original magnification 200×

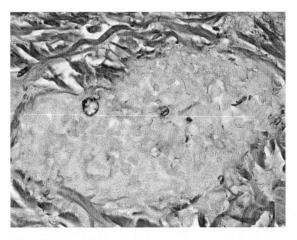

Fig. 2.38 A Warthin–Starry stain demonstrates rare spirochetes, most commonly around vessels in the superficial vascular plexus or along the dermal–epidermal junction. Original magnification 600×

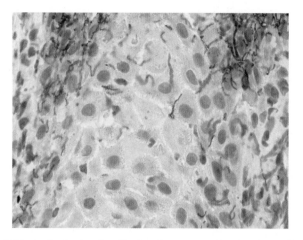

Fig. 2.39 Anti-spirochetal antibodies demonstrate abundant intraepithelial organisms in secondary syphilis. Original magnification 600×

Chapter 3
Superficial Perivascular Dermatitis with Spongiotic Epidermal Changes

- Spongiotic dermatitis

  - Histologic correlate of eczema
  - Presence of edema within the epidermis
  - Superficial perivascular lymphocytic infiltrate
  - Exocytosis of lymphocytes into epidermis
  - Parakeratosis is present except in very acute lesions
  - Infrequent dying keratinocytes
  - Other histologic changes help to subclassify types of spongiotic dermatitis (Figs. 3.1 and 3.2, Table 3.1)

- Allergic contact dermatitis

  - Clinical

    o Erythematous, oozing eruption with small, fragile vesicles
    o May be patterned depending upon contactant
    o Intensely pruritic
    o Overlying scale present in subacute or chronic lesions
    o Results from allergen, such as poison ivy or nickel, contact with previously sensitized skin, i.e., delayed-type hypersensitivity reaction.

  - Histologic

    o Parakeratosis (except in very acute lesions)
    o Increased intercellular edema, or spongiosis

B.R. Smoller, K.M. Hiatt, *Inflammatory Dermatoses: The Basics*,
DOI 10.1007/978-1-4419-6004-7_3,
© Springer Science+Business Media, LLC 2010

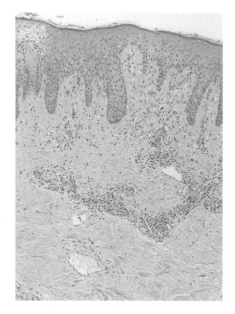

Fig. 3.1 Spongiotic dermatitis is characterized by a superficial perivascular inflammatory infiltrate, exocytosis of lymphocytes, and increased intercellular edema

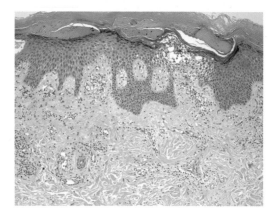

Fig. 3.2 The intercellular edema in spongiotic dermatitis can cause mechanical disruption of the intercellular bridges and result in intraepidermal fluid accumulations, or vesicles

Table 3.1 Spongiotic dermatitis

Allergic contact dermatitis
Irritant contact dermatitis
Nummular dermatitis
Dyshidrotic dermatitis
Pityriasis dermatitis
Seborrheic dermatitis (Volume II, Chapter 4)
Dermatophyte infection
Photo-allergic dermatitis
Id reaction
Gianotti–Crosti syndrome
Bullous pemphigoid, urticarial (Volume II, Chapter 5)
Stasis dermatitis

- o Variable thickening of the epidermis, or acanthosis
- o Exocytosis of lymphocytes and eosinophils into epidermis
- o Langerhans cell microabscesses
- o Rare dying keratinocytes
- o Superficial perivascular infiltrate of lymphocytes and eosinophils
- o Inflammation rarely extends much deeper than superficial vascular plexus
- o Relative abundance of eosinophils may help to distinguish contact dermatitis from other spongiotic dermatoses
- o Photo-allergic drug eruption is histologically identical to allergic contact dermatitis – only distinguishable by history (Figs. 3.3, 3.4, 3.5, and 3.6)

- Irritant contact dermatitis
  - Clinical
    - o Erythematous, oozing eruption, with small vesicles, similar to allergic contact dermatitis
    - o Reaction is limited to sites exposed to irritant
    - o Caused by direct injury to skin from irritants such as alkalis and acids

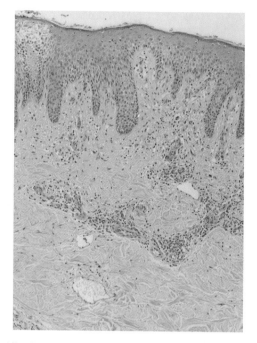

Fig. 3.3 Allergic contact dermatitis shows a spongiotic epidermis with a moderate superficial perivascular lymphocytic infiltrate

- Histology
  - Mixed perivascular inflammatory infiltrate with predominantly lymphocytes and histiocytes, rare neutrophils, and eosinophils accompanied by increased interstitial edema
  - Exocytosis of lymphocytes
  - Increased intercellular edema
  - Scattered dyskeratotic cells which may elicit exocytosis of neutrophils (Fig. 3.7)

- Nummular dermatitis
  - Clinical
    - Coin-sized lesions, most common on trunk and extremities

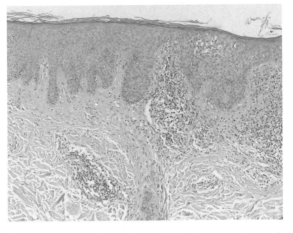

Fig. 3.4 Allergic contact dermatitis, in addition to a spongiotic epidermis, shows increased dermal eosinophils

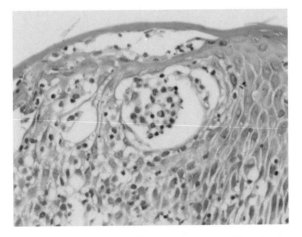

Fig. 3.5 Increased Langerhans cells are seen in the epidermis of spongiotic dermatitides. In this case of allergic contact, these epidermal antigen-presenting cells are forming a microabscess

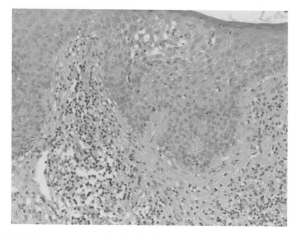

Fig. 3.6 Allergic contact dermatitis shows increased dermal eosinophils, often with exocytosis into the spongiotic epidermis

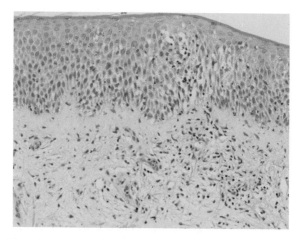

Fig. 3.7 Irritant contact dermatitis show epidermal edema with a superficial perivascular lymphocytic infiltrate. Dyskeratosis of keratinocytes is often seen and this is accompanied by exocytosis of neutrophils, as is seen here

o Intensely pruritic

o Scale in subacute and chronic lesions

– Histologic

o Non-specific changes

o Parakeratosis

o Spongiosis, typically mild

o Variable acanthosis

o Exocytosis of lymphocytes into epidermis

o Eosinophils, typically less abundant than in allergic contact dermatitis

o Superficial perivascular lymphoid infiltrate – relatively mild in most (Figs. 3.8 and 3.9)

• Pompholyx (dyshidrotic dermatitis)

– Clinical

o Erythematous, scaly, and vesicular eruption on hands and feet

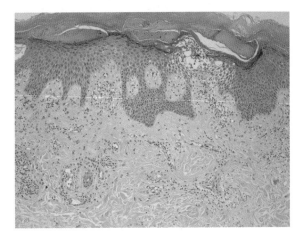

Fig. 3.8 This case of nummular dermatitis shows mild spongiosis with exocytosis of lymphocytes. There is hypergranulosis and hyperkeratosis suggestive of excoriation

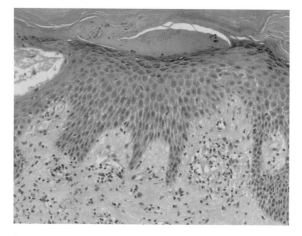

Fig. 3.9 Higher power of the image in Fig. 3.8 shows a mildly spongiotic epidermis with exocytosis of rare lymphocytes, characteristic of nummular dermatitis

- o This is not caused by hyperhidrosis, as originally thought, hence dyshidrotic dermatitis is a discouraged term
- o Exacerbated by cold weather
- o Intensely pruritic

- – Histologic

    - o Spongiosis, often exuberant with vesicle and bullae formation
    - o Exocytosis of lymphocytes into epidermis
    - o Langerhans cell microabscesses
    - o Superficial perivascular lymphoid infiltrate
    - o Rare eosinophils may be present
    - o Almost always on acral skin (Figs. 3.10 and 3.11)

- • Dermatophyte infection

    - – Clinical

        - o Pruritic, erythematous scaly eruption
        - o Most common on trunk, extremities
        - o Uncommon on head and neck of adults

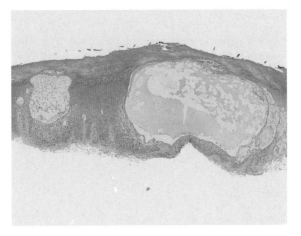

Fig. 3.10 Pompholyx shows variable intraepidermal edema, occasionally forming intraepidermal bullae

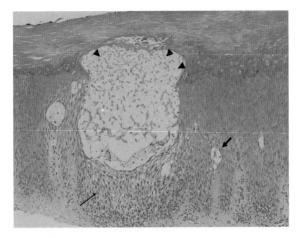

Fig. 3.11 Pompholyx has exocytosis of lymphocytes with spongiosis (*thin arrow*), vesicles (*thick arrow*), and bullae (*arrowheads*)

- Histologic

  - Focal areas of parakeratosis, occasionally with neutrophils in stratum corneum
  - Minimal epidermal spongiosis
  - Exocytosis of lymphocytes
  - Superficial perivascular lymphoid infiltrate, sometimes with admixed neutrophils and/or eosinophils
  - Hyphal and yeast forms observed on PASD or GMS stains (Figs. 3.12, 3.13, and 3.14)

- Pityriasis rosea

  - Clinical

    - Erythematous, scaly, ovoid patches on trunk and proximal extremities – "Christmas tree-like" distribution commonly seen
    - Head and neck usually spared

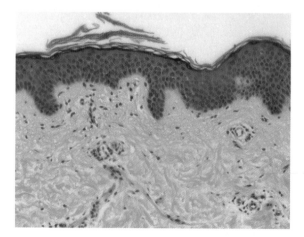

Fig. 3.12 Dermatophytosis shows a superficial perivascular lymphocytic infiltrate, with or without neutrophils, epidermal spongiosis, and focal to exuberant parakeratosis, which may be only focal as in this case

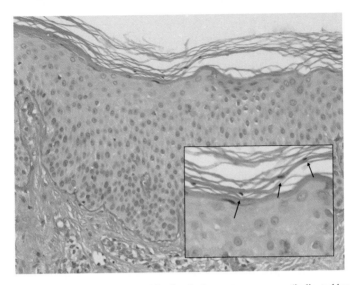

Fig. 3.13 PAS shows the fungal hyphea in the stratum corneum (indicated by *arrows* in inset)

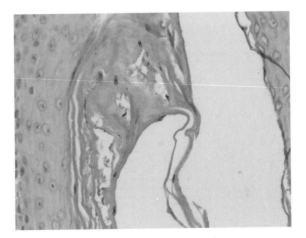

Fig. 3.14 In suspected cases of dermatophytosis, a search in the follicular epithelium may result in finding the hyphae

- o Presents with "herald patch"
- o Seasonal incidences
- o Most common in young adults
- o Resolves spontaneously after 2–3 months

– Histologic

- o Single small tufts of parakeratosis with underlying foci of slight spongiosis
- o Mild exocytosis of lymphocytes
- o Superficial perivascular lymphoid infiltrate
- o Rare eosinophils
- o Hemorrhage within epidermis and papillary dermis (slight)
- o Hemorrhage helps to distinguish from small plaque parapsoriasis (digitate dermatosis) and absence of plasma cells distinguishes from secondary syphilis (Figs. 3.15 and 3.16)

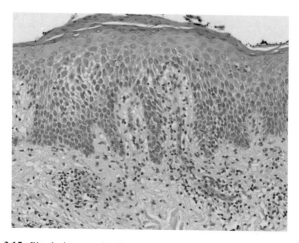

Fig. 3.15 Pityriasis rosea is characterized by tufts of parakeratosis over a spongiotic epidermis

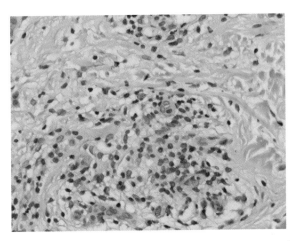

Fig. 3.16 In addition to perivascular lymphocytes, in pityriasis rosea, there is erythrocyte extravasation

- Photo-allergic drug eruption
    - Clinical
        o Allergic reaction to wide range of therapeutic drugs
        o Caused by photosensitivity from a drug metabolite
        o Sun-exposed areas develop an erythematous, vesicular eruption
    - Histologic
        o Indistinguishable from contact dermatitis
        o Distinction made purely upon clinical correlation
        o Irritant contact dermatitis has more dying keratinocytes, fewer eosinophils, and is not particularly spongiotic
        o Photo-toxic drug eruption characterized by dying keratinocytes, lack of eosinophils, and minima spongiosis

- ID reaction
    - Clinical
        o Hypersensitivity reaction to systemic antigen

- No antigen present within the lesions
- Non-specific eczematous patches at any site – resolve with removal of primary antigen

  - Histologic

    - Non-specific features of spongiotic dermatitis with no characteristic changes
    - Cannot make precise diagnosis but only suggest based upon clinical history

- Gianotti–Crosti syndrome

  - Clinical

    - Erythematous papules and patches with overlying scale
    - Most common on extremities, including acral surfaces
    - Associated most commonly with systemic viruses (many associated)
    - No virus actually in lesions – purely hypersensitivity eruption

  - Histologic

    - Non-specific features of spongiotic dermatitis with no characteristic changes
    - Cannot make precise diagnosis but only suggest based upon clinical history

- Other entities that may display a spongiotic dermatitis-like appearance

  - Stasis dermatitis

    - Clinical

      Confined to lower extremities, most common in older adults or those with vascular anomalies
      Erythema, scale, mottled pigmentation
      Dermal sclerosis, loss of appendages
      Bottle-neck deformity when extensive

o Histologic

Non-specific features of spongiotic dermatitis
Main pathologic changes are in the dermis

– Lobular proliferation of thick-walled vessels in papillary (and reticular with more florid cases) dermis

Hemorrhage
Hemosiderin deposition
Dermal sclerosis with loss of appendages in long-standing lesions
Dermal edema may be present
Membranous lipodystrophy (dermatoliposclerosis) sometimes seen in long-standing lesions (Fig. 3.17)

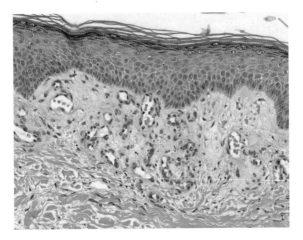

Fig. 3.17 Stasis dermatitis shows spongiosis, overlying a dermal lobular vascular proliferation with erythrocyte extravasation

Chapter 4
Superficial Perivascular Dermatitis with Psoriasiform Epidermal Changes

Clinically, these are papulosquamous disorders (Table 4.1)

Table 4.1 Psoriasiform eruptions

Psoriasis
Seborrheic dermatitis
Secondary syphilis (see also Volume II, Chapter 2)
Lichen simplex chronicus
Pityriasis rubra pilaris
Acrodermatitis enteropathica
Mycosis fungoides (see Volume IV)

- Psoriasis

  - Clinical

    - o Chronic – brown to red papules and plaques
    - o Fine, silvery scale
    - o Auspitz sign – hemorrhage when scale is removed
    - o Koebner phenomenon – psoriasiform lesion arises at the site of trauma
    - o Scalp, acral skin, and extremities usually involved
    - o May progress to diffuse erythroderma
    - o Pustular variant shows less psoriasiform change
    - o Psoriatic arthritis can be crippling

  - Histologic features

    - o Parakeratosis, diffuse, and often thick

B.R. Smoller, K.M. Hiatt, *Inflammatory Dermatoses: The Basics*,
DOI 10.1007/978-1-4419-6004-7_4,
© Springer Science+Business Media, LLC 2010

- o Loss or diminution of granular layer (only partial with guttate lesions)
- o Munro microabscesses (collections of neutrophils within the stratum corneum)
- o Spongiform pustule of Kogoj (collections of neutrophils within the upper portions of the epidermis)
- o Psoriasiform hyperplasia (regular elongation of rete ridges)
- o Suprapapillary thinning
- o Minimal spongiosis
- o Ectatic papillary dermal blood vessels
- o Mild superficial perivascular lymphoid infiltrate
- o Minimal eosinophils or plasma cells
- o Deep inflammation very uncommon
- o Pustular variant has markedly different histologic changes

Subcorneal neutrophilic abscess
Minimal psoriasiform epidermal hyperplasia
No parakeratosis
Focal spongiosis
No suprapapillary thinning (Figs. 4.1, 4.2, 4.3, 4.4, and 4.5)

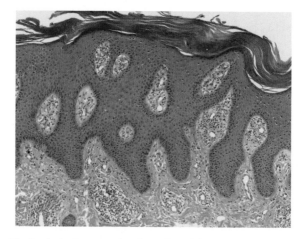

Fig. 4.1 Psoriasis shows regular elongation of the rete with thinning of the suprapapillary plate. There is also loss of the granular cell layer and confluent, often thick, parakeratosis

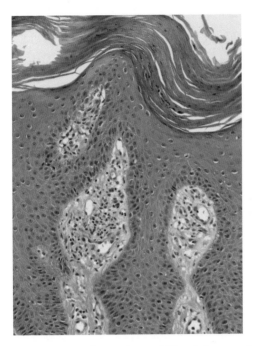

Fig. 4.2 This higher power image shows additional features of psoriasis, including the neutrophilic infiltrate that extends into the stratum corneum (Munro microabscess) and tortuous ectatic vessels in the papillary dermis

- Seborrheic dermatitis

  - Clinical

    o Sharply defined red-brown patches with fine scaling
    o May resemble psoriasis
    o Oozing may be present, but no vesicles
    o Usually on scalp, face (perinasal), chest
    o "Dandruff" is seborrheic dermatitis

  - Histologic features

    o Parakeratosis
    o Psoriasiform epidermal hyperplasia

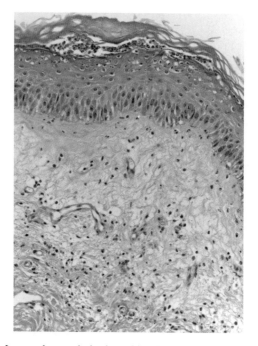

Fig. 4.3 In pustular psoriasis the epidermis does not show psoriasiform hyperplasia. Parakeratosis is not evident and there may be some retention of the granular cells layer. Notably, however, the neutrophilic exudate is pronounced

- o Perifollicular spongiosis (mild)
- o Neutrophils present at follicular orifices
- o Mild superficial perivascular lymphoid infiltrate
- o No suprapapillary thinning
- o Granular layer preserved
- o Differentiate from psoriasis based upon folliculocentric nature of process, retention of granular layer, follicular spongiosis (Figs. 4.6 and 4.7)

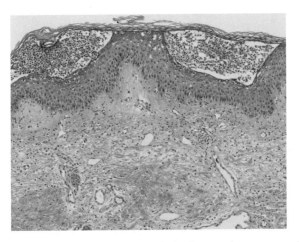

Fig. 4.4 Some cases of pustular psoriasis show exuberant neutrophilic exocytosis in the stratum corneum with pronounced subcorneal abscesses

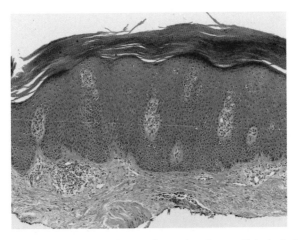

Fig. 4.5 Guttate psoriasis is a subtype based on clinical findings. Histologically, there is focal psoriasiform epidermal hyperplasia with loss of the granular cell layer, exocytosis of neutrophils, and confluent parakeratosis

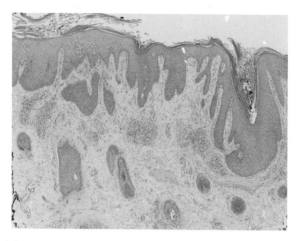

Fig. 4.6 Seborrheic dermatitis shows epidermal hyperplasia, parakeratosis, spongiosis, and exocytosis of neutrophils

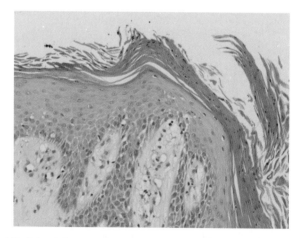

Fig. 4.7 Seborrheic dermatitis is characterized by folliculocentric changes of epithelial hyperplasia, spongiosis, and parakeratosis

- Secondary syphilis

  - Clinical features

    - Great mimicker
    - Most commonly resembles pityriasis rosea
    - Erythematous macules or patches on trunk, extremities, especially involving palms and soles
    - Can also resemble guttate psoriasis
    - Mucous patches are present and condyloma lata are specific
    - Ulceration is very rare

  - Histologic features

    - Psoriasiform epidermal hyperplasia
    - No suprapapillary thinning
    - Granular layer is preserved
    - Lichenoid and deeper perivascular infiltrate of lymphocytes with scattered plasma cells
    - Endothelial cell swelling – not specific
    - Difficult to find organisms with Warthin–Starry stains in secondary syphilis

      Usually along the dermal–epidermal junction or around superficial vascular plexus blood vessels

    - Anti-spirochetal antibodies far more sensitive (Figs. 4.8, 4.9, and 4.10)

- Lichen simplex chronicus (formerly known as neurodermatitis)

  - Clinical features

    - Area of chronic, persistent rubbing
    - Intensely pruritic patches and/or plaques
    - Often on extensor surfaces of extremities but can be anywhere
    - Prurigo nodularis – closely related, but with a nodular configuration

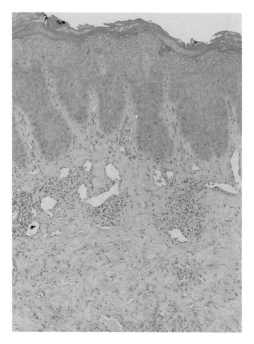

Fig. 4.8 Secondary syphilis shows epidermal hyperplasia, with retention of the granular cell layer and no suprapapillary thinning

- Histologic features

  o Hyperkeratosis, occasional parakeratosis
  o Psoriasiform epidermal hyperplasia
  o Hypergranulosis
  o Papillary dermal fibrosis
  o No suprapapillary thinning
  o Minimal inflammation in most cases
  o Epidermis appears acral even though dermis demonstrates appendages and other features of non-acral skin (Fig. 4.11)

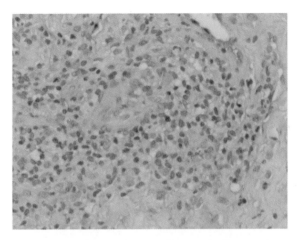

Fig. 4.9 Endothelial hyperplasia and a perivascular infiltrate with numerous plasma cells, as noted in this case, are classic but not always seen

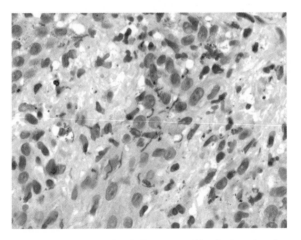

Fig. 4.10 Anti-spirochete antibody is very sensitive in detecting the organisms in syphilis (anti-spirochete antibody, 600×)

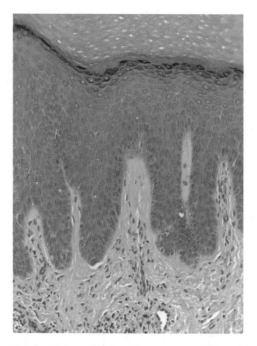

Fig. 4.11 Lichen simplex chronicus shows an acanthotic epidermis with hypergranulosis, hyperkeratosis, and a thick suprapapillary plate. The dermis characteristically shows vertical orientation of the papillary dermal collagen and a minimal superficial perivascular lymphocytic infiltrate

- Pityriasis rubra pilaris

  - Clinical

    ○ Childhood and adult variants
    ○ Often starts with perifollicular, hyperkeratotic papules
    ○ Spreads to be almost erythrodermic, with large islands of sparing
    ○ Dorsum of hands frequently involved with follicular papules

  - Histologic features

    ○ Hyperkeratosis

- o Parakeratosis confined to shoulders of follicular ostia
- o Psoriasiform epidermal hyperplasia (blunted)
- o Granular layer is preserved
- o Rare acantholytic cells
- o Mild superficial perivascular lymphocytic infiltrate without eosinophils or plasma cells
- o Slight exocytosis
- o Subtle and difficult histologic diagnosis
- o Usually less inflammatory than psoriasis (Fig. 4.12)

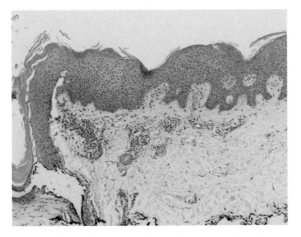

Fig. 4.12 The epidermal hyperplasia in pityriasis rubra pilaris is incomplete. Parakeratosis is patchy with prevalence for the follicular ostium. There is preservation of the granular cell layer

- • Acrodermatitis enteropathica

    - – Clinical

        - o Associated with zinc deficiency
        - o Acral and perioral site predominance
        - o Erythematous, scaly eruption

    - – Histologic features

        - o Confluent parakeratosis

- ○ Absent granular cell layer
- ○ Epidermal hyperplasia
- ○ Mild spongiosis with exocytosis of lymphocytes
- ○ Individual acantholysis may become confluent causing intraepidermal vesicles and bullae (Fig. 4.13)

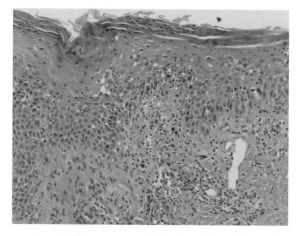

Fig. 4.13 Acrodermatitis enteropathica shows variable acanthosis, absent granular cell layer, and confluent parakeratosis. Spongiosis is accompanied by exocytosis of lymphocytes, and characteristically, there is acantholysis that may become confluent

Chapter 5
Superepidermal Blistering Processes

- Bullous diseases

  Histologically characterized by location of the blister and further by the associated inflammatory infiltrate, or lack of.

  – Subepidermal
  – Intraepidermal

    o Intrabasilar
    o Suprabasilar
    o Mid-epidermal
    o Subcorneal

- Subepidermal blisters

  – Non-inflammatory (Table 5.1)
  – Inflammatory

    o Lymphohistiocytic infiltrate
    o Eosinophils predominate
    o Neutrophils predominate
    o Mast cells predominate

Table 5.1 Subepidermal blisters – non-inflammatory

Epidermolysis bullosa – junctional and dystrophic subtypes
Porphyria cutanea tarda
Bullous pemphigoid (cell-poor variant)

B.R. Smoller, K.M. Hiatt, *Inflammatory Dermatoses: The Basics*,
DOI 10.1007/978-1-4419-6004-7_5,
© Springer Science+Business Media, LLC 2010

- Epidermolysis bullosa

  - Very rare
  - Hereditary mechanical blistering process
  - Most children born with blisters
  - Level of blister determines clinical course and prognosis

    - Dystrophic
    - Junctional
    - Simplex (not subepidermal) – see intraepidermal blistering disorders

- Epidermolysis bullosa – dystrophic

  - Clinical

    - Worst prognosis – inherited autosomal recessive (worse) or autosomal dominant (attenuated form)
    - Blisters heal with scarring
    - Fusion of fingers and toes
    - Joint contractures
    - Eyelids fuse
    - Similar processes in esophagus
    - Predisposition to develop squamous cell carcinoma of skin
    - Markedly shortened life expectancy

  - Histologic

    - Split occurs deep to the lamina densa
    - Caused by decreased numbers of anchoring fibrils (type VII collagen)
    - No keratinocyte necrosis present in acute blisters
    - No inflammation present in acute blisters
    - Precise diagnosis usually requires electron microscopy or immunofluorescence to detect aberrant basement membrane protein expression (Figs. 5.1 and 5.2)

- Epidermolysis bullosa – junctional

  - Clinical

    - Several variants – most common is autosomal recessively inherited

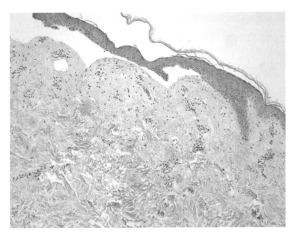

Fig. 5.1 Dystrophic epidermolysis bullosa demonstrates a non-inflammatory subepidermal blister. Original magnification 100×

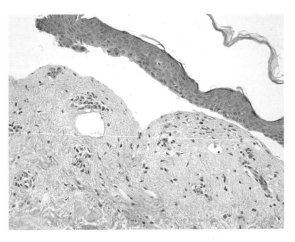

Fig. 5.2 The subepidermal blister in epidermolysis bullosa is caused by mechanical disruption of the basement membrane zone due to structural anomalies. Thus, no keratinocyte necrosis is identified. Original magnification 200×

  o Some variants fatal, others with good prognosis
  o Pyloric atresia associated with some subtypes
  o Prognosis related to deficient structural protein leading to
     blistering process

 – Histologic

  o Split is between basal keratinocyte and lamina lucida
  o On electron microscopy, loss of hemidesmosomes is
     apparent – usually required for diagnosis of precise
     subtype
  o Desmosomes (between keratinocytes) are uninvolved
  o No keratinocyte necrosis present in acute blisters
  o No inflammation present in acute blisters (Fig. 5.3)

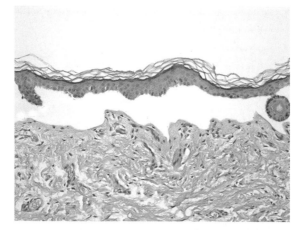

Fig. 5.3 Histologic findings in junctional type of epidermolysis bullosa also
demonstrate a non-inflammatory subepidermal blister similar to that seen in
the dystrophic subtype. Original magnification 100×

• Porphyria cutanea tarda

 – Clinical

  o Reduced uroporphyrinogen decarboxylase activity

- o Can be inherited (autosomal dominant) or sporadic (associated most commonly with alcoholic liver disease or hepatitis C)
- o Small vesicles on dorsal hands, face, and arms
- o Also see milia, scarring, hypertrichosis
- o Associated with higher incidence of hepatocellular carcinoma

– Histologic

- o Non-inflammatory subepidermal blister
- o Marked solar elastosis in most cases
- o Perivascular deposition of eosinophilic material causes vessels to remain widely patent on routine sections (PAS positive)
- o Thick-walled papillary dermal vessels lead to festooning – preservation of papillary dermal tip architecture underneath blister cavity
- o "Caterpillar bodies" – basement membrane material and dying keratinocytes are present within the epidermis (Figs. 5.4, 5.5, 5.6, and 5.7, Table 5.2)

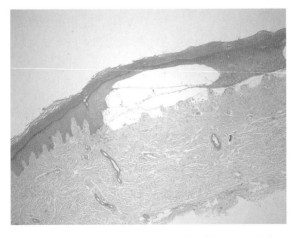

Fig. 5.4 Porphyria cutanea tarda is characterized by a non-inflammatory subepidermal blister, often on acral skin. Original magnification 40×

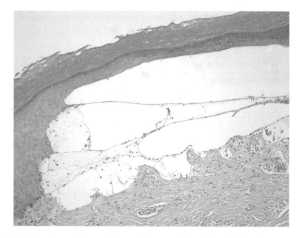

Fig. 5.5 Prominent festooning of the papillary dermal tips is caused by thickened dermal blood vessel walls in porphyria cutanea tarda. Original magnification 200×

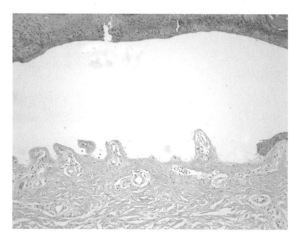

Fig. 5.6 Thickened vessel walls can usually be seen with routine staining in porphyria cutanea tarda. Original magnification 100×

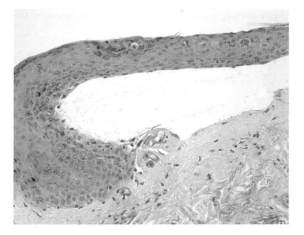

Fig. 5.7 In some cases, PAS stains are helpful in demonstrating the vascular wall thickening in porphyria cutanea tarda. Original magnification 200×. Periodic acid Schiff stain

Table 5.2   Subepidermal blisters – lymphohistiocytic infiltrate

Erythema multiforme (and variants – see Volume II, Chapter 2)
Lichen sclerosus (see Volume II, Chapter 2)
Lichen planus (see Volume II, Chapter 4)
Polymorphous light eruption (also in Volume II, Chapter 1)

- Polymorphous light eruption

  - Clinical

    o Occurs following initial exposure to sun each year and abates within 1–2 weeks
    o So-called hardening or tolerance to sun exposure occurs each year during summer months and lesions recur following winter in most cases
    o Uncommon near equator, not infrequent in more temperate climates
    o Papules, urticarial plaques, vesicles on sun-exposed sites (polymorphous)
    o Usually occurs in young adults (3rd and 4th decades)

   o UV-A appears to be the main causative agent (also UV-B
      to lesser degree)

 – Histologic

   o Superficial and deep perivascular lymphocytic infiltrate –
      rare eosinophils in some cases
   o Minimal epidermal changes – occasionally slight
      spongiosis
   o Often (but not always) marked papillary dermal edema
   o Mucin is not present (in contrast to lupus erythematosus)
   o Direct immunofluorescence essentially negative (Figs.
      5.8, 5.9, and 5.10, Table 5.3)

• Bullous pemphigoid

 – Occurs most commonly in elderly patients
 – Good prognosis

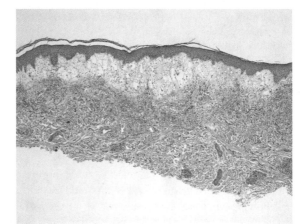

Fig. 5.8 Polymorphous light eruption (PMLE) is characterized by a subepidermal blister caused by massive papillary dermal edema. There is also a
superficial and deep perivascular, almost exclusively lymphocytic inflammatory infiltrate. Original magnification 40×

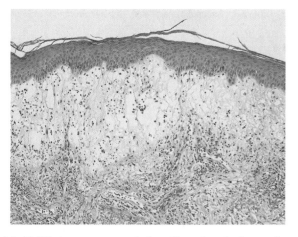

Fig. 5.9 PMLE demonstrates marked papillary dermal edema, often with little overlying spongiosis. Original magnification 100×

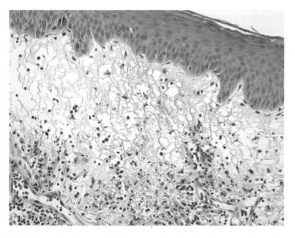

Fig. 5.10 The subepidermal blister seen in PMLE is caused solely by the dermal edema, and no keratinocyte necrosis is identified. This is in contrast to lupus erythematosus that has some similar histologic features, but also demonstrates basal cell necrosis. Original magnification 200×

Table 5.3 Subepidermal blisters – eosinophilic infiltrate

Bullous pemphigoid
Pemphigoides (herpes) gestationis
Bullous arthropod bite (see Volume II, Chapter 1)
Bullous drug eruption (see Volume II, Chapter 1)

– Purported relationship with internal malignancy probably not real
– Clinical features

   o Large, tense blisters in groin, axilla, flexors of extremities
   o Blisters rapidly heal when broken, without scarring
   o Surrounding erythema may be present

– Histologic

   o Subepidermal split
   o Eosinophils and lymphocytes in blister cavity and superficial dermis
   o Eosinophilic microabscesses in dermal papillae in some cases
   o Spongiosis abundant, but no necrosis (except in older lesions) (Figs. 5.11, 5.12, 5.13, and 5.14)

– Histogenesis

   o Split in mid-lamina lucida
   o Autoantibody directed against one of the two bullous pemphigoid antigens

      BP I – 180 kDa – wholly within lamina lucida
      BP II – 230 kDa – transcends lamina lucida into lower portion of basal keratinocyte

   o Mast cell degranulation
   o Eosinophil chemotaxis

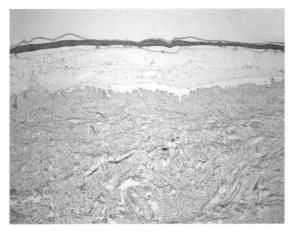

Fig. 5.11 Bullous pemphigoid (BP) is characterized by a neat subepidermal blister and usually has abundant inflammatory cells within and below the blister cavity. Original magnification 40×

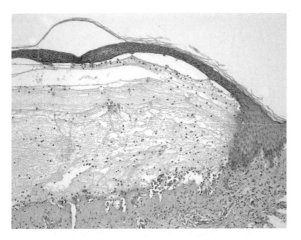

Fig. 5.12 The edge of the blister demonstrates an inflammatory process, but with no keratinocyte necrosis in BP. Original magnification 100×

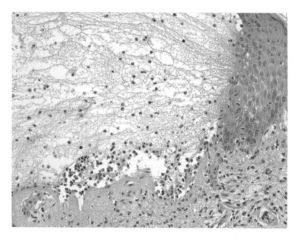

Fig. 5.13 In most cases of BP, the inflammatory infiltrate consists of primarily eosinophils. Original magnification 200×

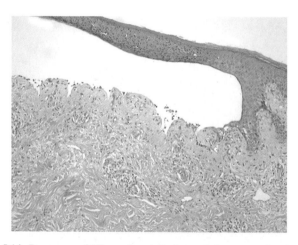

Fig. 5.14 Rare cases of BP may be relatively non-inflammatory but demonstrate the neat subepidermal blister. Original magnification 100×

- Direct immunofluorescence

  o Linear IgG and C3 along dermal–epidermal junction (same pattern independent of autoantigen as described above)
  o IgA and IgM may be present less frequently
  o DIF performed on "salt-split skin" reveals antibodies on roof of blister (*in contrast to epidermolysis bullosa acquisita that has the same autoantibodies but located on the floor of the blister cavity*) (Figs. 5.15 and 5.16)

- Indirect immunofluorescence – positive in about 70% of active cases

• Pemphigoides (herpes) gestationis

  - Clinical

    o No relationship to herpes virus!
    o "Bullous pemphigoid of pregnancy"
    o Uncommon
    o Occurs in final two trimesters of pregnancy

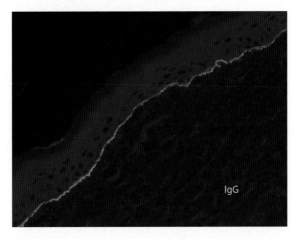

Fig. 5.15 Direct immunofluorescence demonstrates linear staining along the basement membrane zone with IgG (seen here) and C3. Original magnification 100×

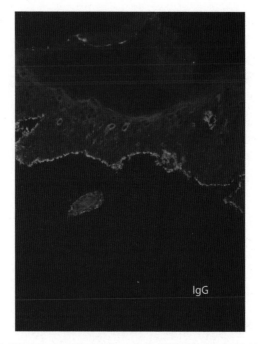

Fig. 5.16 Direct immunofluorescence performed on "salt-split" skin reveals linear deposits of IgG along the roof of the separation (directed against the bullous pemphigoid antigen located in the lamina lucida). Original magnification 100×

- ○ Recurrences common with subsequent pregnancies and may be more intense disease with earlier onset
- ○ Tense blisters with erythema
- ○ Very pruritic
- ○ Purported relationship with increased fetal mortality now largely disproven

- – Histologic

  - ○ Subepidermal blister
  - ○ Spongiosis
  - ○ Rare necrotic keratinocytes in some cases (unlike BP)
  - ○ Eosinophils along dermal–epidermal junction and superficial dermis (Figs. 5.17 and 5.18)

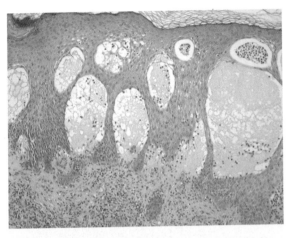

Fig. 5.17 Pemphigoides gestationis (PG, herpes gestationis) is characterized by an inflammatory subepidermal blister. Original magnification 100×

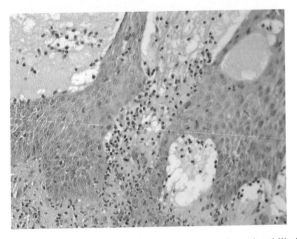

Fig. 5.18 In most cases of HG, there is a predominantly eosinophilic infiltrate. Distinction from bullous pemphigoid is made primarily based upon clinical history. Original magnification 200×

– Direct immunofluorescence

  ○ Linear C3 at dermal–epidermal junction
  ○ Linear IgG along dermal–epidermal junction found in
    <50% of cases
  ○ Most cases fail to demonstrate immunoglobulin deposi-
    tion (Fig. 5.19 and Table 5.4)

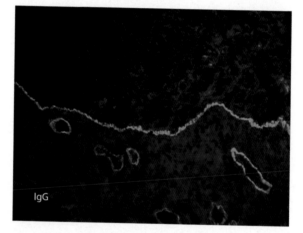

Fig. 5.19 The direct immunofluorescence staining pattern in pemphigoides gestationis is similar to that seen in bullous pemphigoid with linear deposits of IgG (demonstrated here) and C3 along the basement membrane zone. Original magnification 100×

Table 5.4 Subepidermal blister – neutrophilic infiltrate

Dermatitis herpetiformis
Linear IgA bullous dermatosis of childhood
Linear IgA bullous dermatosis
Cicatricial pemphigoid
Bullous lupus erythematosus (see Volume II, Chapter 2)
Leukocytoclastic vasculitis (see Volume II, Chapter 8)

• Dermatitis herpetiformis

  – Clinical

    ○ Intensely pruritic

- o Symmetrical papules and vesicles
- o Extensor surfaces of extremities (especially knees, elbows)
- o Sacral involvement
- o Usually arises early in adult life
- o Associated with small intestinal villous atrophy in all cases
- o Most patients have subclinical features of celiac sprue
- o Long-standing untreated disease associated with high-grade gastrointestinal lymphomas

- Histologic features

- o Subepidermal blister (usually very small – confined to 1–2 rete ridges)
- o Neutrophilic abscesses in dermal papillae
- o Perivascular infiltrate of *lymphocytes* around superficial vascular plexus
- o No keratinocyte necrosis (Figs. 5.20 and 5.21)

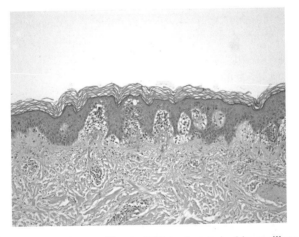

Fig. 5.20 Dermatitis herpetiformis (DH) is characterized by papillary dermal microabscesses that result in very small subepidermal vesicles. Original magnification 100×

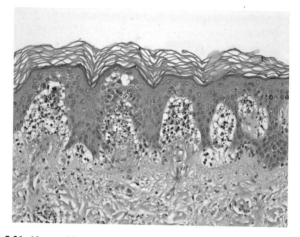

Fig. 5.21 Neutrophils comprise the cellular infiltrate within the papillary dermal tips in DH. Original magnification 200×

- Direct immunofluorescence

    ○ Granular deposits of IgA in papillary dermal tips

        Resembles "snow-capped mountains"

    ○ Lesional skin usually negative – consumption of immunoglobulins by neutrophils (speculative) (Fig. 5.22)

- Linear IgA bullous dermatosis

    - Histologically identical to bullous dermatosis of childhood (also identical immunofluorescence findings)
    - Most commonly related to drug exposure

        ○ Vancomycin is the most frequent association in in-patient setting

    - Bullous dermatosis of childhood not related to drug exposure
    - Clinical

        ○ Large tense blisters on trunk and extremities
        ○ Pruritic
        ○ Can form annular configuration with blisters at periphery

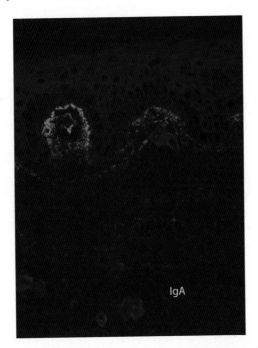

Fig. 5.22 Direct immunofluorescence demonstrates granular deposits of IgA within the papillary dermal tips in peri-lesional skin. Original magnification 200×

- Histologic
    o Large subepidermal split (in contrast to small splits seen in dermatitis herpetiformis)
    o Abundant neutrophils linearly arrayed along dermal–epidermal junction
    o Rare eosinophils may be present
    o Dying keratinocytes unusual (Figs. 5.23, 5.24, and 5.25)

- Direct immunofluorescence
    o Linear deposits along dermal–epidermal junction with IgA and C3
    o *Deposits in DH are granular and discontinuous* (Fig. 5.26)

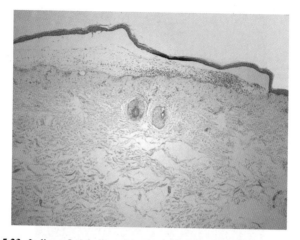

Fig. 5.23 In linear IgA bullous dermatosis (LABD) the subepidermal blister is much larger than that seen in dermatitis herpetiformis. Original magnification 40×

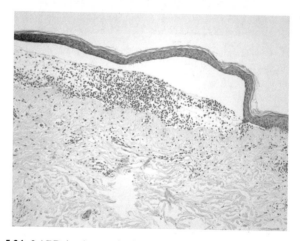

Fig. 5.24 LABD is characterized by a pronounced neutrophilic infiltrate within and below the blister cavity and lack of keratinocyte necrosis. Original magnification 100×

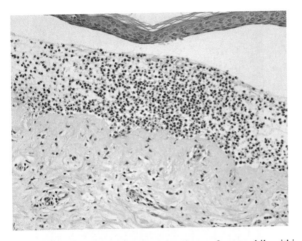

Fig. 5.25 In LABD, there are often extensive sheets of neutrophils within and below the subepidermal blister. Original magnification 200×

- Cicatricial pemphigoid

    - Clinical

        o Blistering occurs most commonly on mucosal surfaces of older patients
        o More common in women
        o Oral ulcerations in up to 85%
        o Persistent disease can result in blindness if there is ocular involvement
        o May occur exclusively on skin surfaces without mucosal involvement
        o Some association with internal malignancy, autoimmune processes

    - Histologic

        o Subepidermal blister
        o No necrosis of overlying keratinocytes
        o Mixed infiltrate of inflammatory cells in dermis or submucosa

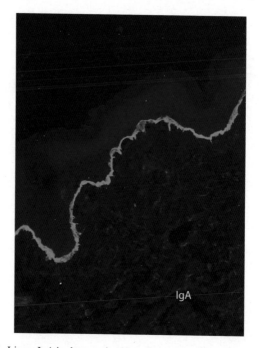

Fig. 5.26 Linear IgA is characterized by a linear deposition of IgA (seen here) and C3 along the dermal–epidermal junction. Original magnification 100×

- ○ Includes majority of neutrophils in most cases, but significant numbers of eosinophils, lymphocytes (and plasma cells on mucosal surfaces)
- ○ Deeper biopsies may reveal areas of dermal fibrosis and scar formation
- ○ Direct immunofluorescence demonstrates IgG and C3 along the dermal–epidermal junction in a linear pattern – IgA less commonly present (Figs. 5.27 and 5.28)

- – Pathogenesis

  - ○ Heterogeneous group of autoimmune diseases with antibodies directed against various components of the

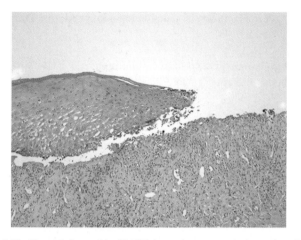

Fig. 5.27 Cicatricial pemphigoid (CP) is most common on mucosal surfaces and results in inflammatory submucosal blisters. Original magnification 100×

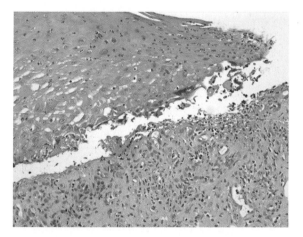

Fig. 5.28 Neutrophils are predominant, but the infiltrate is mixed in CP. Original magnification 200×

dermal–epidermal junction including epiligrin (laminin 5) and BP180

- Subepidermal blister – mast cell infiltrate
- Bullous urticaria pigmentosa and mastocytoma

  - Clinical

    o May be systemic or localized to skin
    o Can occur in pediatric population or in adults
    o May be sporadic or inherited in an autosomal dominant manner
    o Childhood forms usually clear at puberty, lack systemic involvement
    o Associated with flushing, palpitations, diarrhea
    o Maculopapular eruption known as telangiectasia macularis eruptiva perstans (most common, usually in adults) – does not usually cause subepidermal blisters
    o Bullae and nodules (children, usually seen with mastocytomas)
    o Diffuse erythroderma
    o When mast cell disease occurs in adults, it may be associated with bone marrow involvement (mast cell leukemia) and requires systemic workup

  - Histologic

    o Spongiosis
    o Subepidermal split secondary to massive localized edema
    o Abundant mast cells
    o Basal cell hyperpigmentation
    o CD117 (c-kit) or mast cell tryptase immunostains helpful in identifying mast cells
    o Telangiectasia macularis eruptiva perstans variant with increased mast cells admixed with lymphocytes
    o Mastocytomas with sheets of dermal mast cells (Figs. 5.29, 5.30 and 5.31)

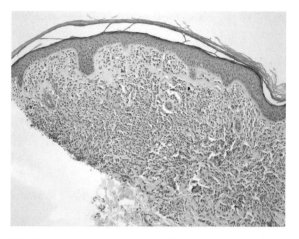

Fig. 5.29 Mastocytomas are characterized by dense sheets of mast cells within the dermis, often resulting in marked papillary dermal edema and subepidermal blister formation. Original magnification 100×

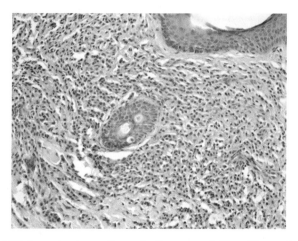

Fig. 5.30 In mastocytomas, the mast cells are remarkably uniform, cuboidal cells with central nuclei and abundant eosinophilic cytoplasm. Original magnification 200×

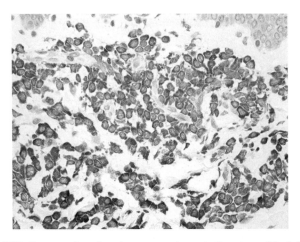

Fig. 5.31 In cases where there is some question as to the nature of the inflammatory infiltrate, Giemsa stains are very helpful in eliciting a metachromatic cytoplasmic stain within mast cells. Original magnification 400×

Chapter 6
Intraepidermal Blisters

- Intrabasilar blisters

  - Epidermolysis bullosa simplex

- Epidermolysis bullosa simplex

  - Clinical

    o Many variants
    o All with favorable prognosis
    o Autosomal dominant inheritance in most cases
    o All variants tend to improve with age
    o Fragile blisters most common at sites of repeated trauma (acral)
    o Blisters heal with minimal to no scarring, occasional milia formation

  - Histologic

    o Split within basal keratinocytes (subnuclear)
    o No inflammation
    o On routine sections may appear subepidermal or may see residuum of basal keratinocyte cytoplasm at the base of the blister
    o Due to abnormal production/clumping of cytokeratins 5 and 14

B.R. Smoller, K.M. Hiatt, *Inflammatory Dermatoses: The Basics*,   107
DOI 10.1007/978-1-4419-6004-7_6,
© Springer Science+Business Media, LLC 2010

o Often requires electron microscopy to precisely subclassify subtype (Fig. 6.1, Table 6.1)

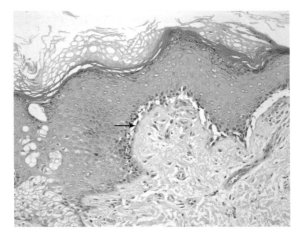

Fig. 6.1 Epidermolysis bullosa demonstrates a separation within the lower half of the basal keratinocytes. The *arrow* points to basal keratinocyte cytoplasm located on the floor of the blister in this case. On routine sectioning, this may often appear to be subepidermal. Original magnification 200×

Table 6.1 Suprabasilar blisters

Pemphigus vulgaris
Pemphigus vegetans
Paraneoplastic pemphigus
Hailey-Hailey (benign familial pemphigus)
Darier's disease (keratosis follicularis)
Grover's disease (transient acantholytic dermatosis)
Warty dyskeratoma
Actinic keratoses (see Volume III, Keratinocytic Neoplasms)

- Pemphigus vulgaris

  - Clinical

    o Flaccid bullae that break easily resulting in extensive denudation (+ Nikolsky sign)

- o Usually in elderly
- o Oral lesions common (>80% of cases)
- o Mortality rate diminished with steroids and other steroid-sparing regimens
- o Autoimmune process

- Histologic

  - o Acantholysis is the main requirement
  - o Suprabasilar split with acantholysis of roof
  - o "Tombstoning" appearance of basal layer keratinocytes
  - o Eosinophils often present in sparse inflammatory response (Figs. 6.2 and 6.3)

- Pathogenesis

  - o Autoimmune process
  - o Autoantibodies directed against desmoglein III
  - o Direct immunofluorescence demonstrates IgG and C3 surrounding keratinocytes (chicken wire pattern)

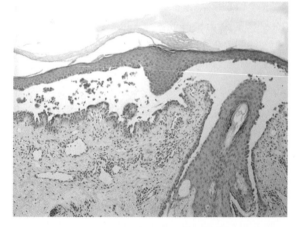

Fig. 6.2 Pemphigus vulgaris is characterized by a suprabasilar split with a row of basal keratinocytes remaining on the floor of the blister cavity. Original magnification 100×

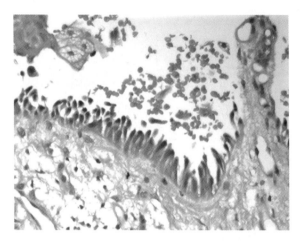

Fig. 6.3 In pemphigus vulgaris, dissolution of the desmosomes by autoantibodies and retention of the hemidesmosomes result in a "tombstone"-like appearance along the basal layer. Original magnification 100×

  o Indirect immunofluorescence with similar pattern – titers can be used to monitor progress of disease (Fig. 6.4)

• Pemphigus vegetans

  – Rare variant of pemphigus vulgaris (perhaps occurring in patients with increased resistance to the process)
  – Lesions are hyperkeratotic and verrucous, difficult to find blisters
  – Histologic

    o Pseudoepitheliomatous hyperplasia
    o Acantholysis (subtle)
    o Eosinophilic microabscesses (Fig. 6.5)

• Paraneoplastic pemphigus

  – Clinical

    o Painful oral ulcerations present in virtually all patients
    o Involvement of other mucosal surfaces (including bronchi) not uncommon

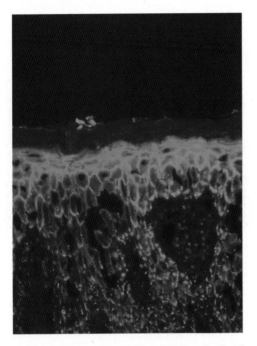

Fig. 6.4 Direct immunofluorescence with anti-IgG antibodies demonstrates a "chicken wire" pattern surrounding keratinocytes in pemphigus vulgaris. Original magnification 100×

- o Flaccid blisters similar to those seen in pemphigus vulgaris also seen
- o Some patients develop lesions more similar to those seen in lichen planus
- o May antedate or coincide with presentation of systemic process
- o Associated with internal malignancies, especially hematologic
- o Also associated with Castleman's disease
- o Most commonly, lesions of paraneoplastic pemphigus resolve as the underlying illness is put into remission

 – Histologic

- o Suprabasilar acantholysis resulting in small blisters – often difficult to find characteristic areas

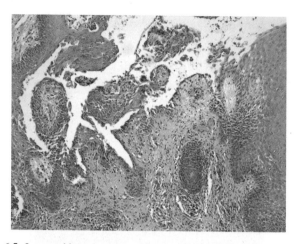

Fig. 6.5 In pemphigus vegetans, there is epidermal hyperplasia in addition to acantholysis. Eosinophilic microabscesses are often seen. Original magnification 100×

- ○ Lichenoid or interface dermatitis with scattered dying keratinocytes *(different from that seen in pemphigus vulgaris)*
- ○ Scattered eosinophils in superficial dermis (Figs. 6.6 and 6.7)

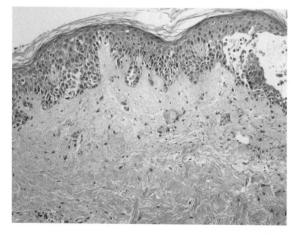

Fig. 6.6 Paraneoplastic pemphigus is characterized by acantholysis, basal vacuolization, and occasional dying keratinocytes with a variably intense lymphocytic infiltrate. Original magnification 100×

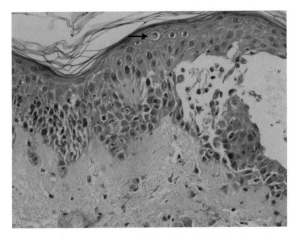

Fig. 6.7 Exocytosis of lymphocytes, rare dying keratinocytes (*arrow*), and focal acantholysis are seen in paraneoplastic pemphigus, making the diagnosis difficult on routine sections. Original magnification 200×

- Pathogenesis

  o Autoantibodies directed against envoplakin and periplakin portions of desmosomal plaques
  o Autoantibodies may be produced by neoplastic cells
  o Indirect immunofluorescence demonstrates similar "chicken wire" staining pattern with IgG and C3 as is seen in pemphigus vulgaris, *but* requires mouse bladder as substrate for maximum sensitivity

- Hailey-Hailey disease

  - Clinical

    o Autosomal dominant
    o Small, flaccid vesicles on erythematous base
    o Mainly in axillae and groin
    o "Wet", macerated lesions
    o Mucosa not usually involved

- Histologic

  ○ Suprabasilar blister (irregular level of separation within epidermis)
  ○ Acantholysis and *corps ronds* not very prominent
  ○ "Dilapidated brick wall" appearance of roof of blister
  ○ Blister extends quite broadly
  ○ Prominent spongiosis
  ○ Mixed inflammatory infiltrate (Figs. 6.8 and 6.9)

- Pathogenesis

  ○ Mutation in *ATP2C1* gene
  ○ Abnormal keratinization
  ○ Direct immunofluorescence – negative
  ○ Not an autoimmune process

• Darier's disease

  - Clinical

    ○ Autosomal dominant

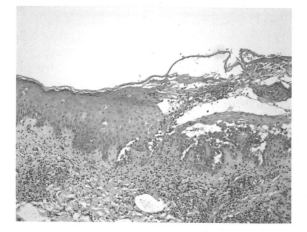

Fig. 6.8 In Hailey-Hailey disease, the suprabasilar blister extends broadly and is accompanied by spongiosis and an inflammatory infiltrate. Original magnification 100×

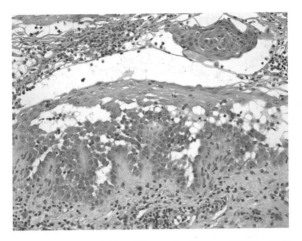

Fig. 6.9 A "dilapidated brick" wall is seen in this case of Hailey-Hailey disease as evidenced by the dissolving roof of the blister. Original magnification 200×

- o Slowly progressive, verrucous, markedly hyperkeratotic lesions in seborrheic distribution
- o Can be very extensive and malodorous
- o Associated with acrokeratosis verruciformis of Hopf (on wrists)

- Histologic

    - o Marked overlying hyperkeratosis – usually orthokeratotic
    - o Dyskeratosis resulting in *corps ronds* and *grains*
    - o Suprabasilar acantholysis
    - o Dermal papillae lined by single layer of basal keratinocytes (pseudovillus formation)
    - o Lymphoid infiltrate – mildly intense (Figs. 6.10, 6.11, and 6.12)

- Pathogenesis

    - o Abnormal keratinization
    - o Mutation in *ATP2A2* gene
    - o Direct immunofluorescence – negative
    - o Not an autoimmune process

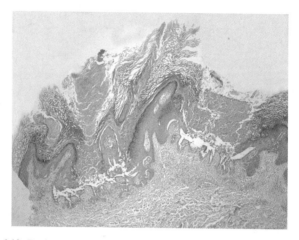

Fig. 6.10 Darier's disease demonstrates marked hyperkeratosis overlying the suprabasilar blister caused by acantholysis. Original magnification 40×

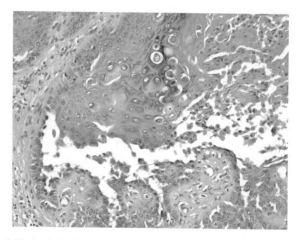

Fig. 6.11 Darier's disease demonstrates a suprabasilar blister, often with elongated rete ridges, *corps ronds* and *grains*, and dense hyperkeratosis. Original magnification 200×

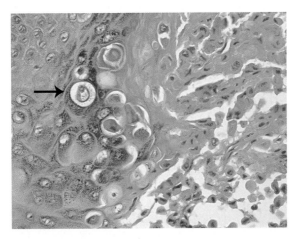

Fig. 6.12 Prominent *corps ronds* (*arrow*) and *grains* are seen in Darier's disease. Original magnification 400×

- Grover's disease

    - Clinical

        o Intensely pruritic tiny vesicles and papules on chest, back, thighs
        o Middle-aged to elderly men
        o Can last weeks to years

    - Histologic

        o No specific pattern
        o Histologic changes can mimic

            Pemphigus vulgaris
            Darier's disease
            Hailey-Hailey disease
            Pemphigus foliaceus
            Spongiotic dermatitis

        o May have several patterns in tiny regions
        o Clinical correlation essential for making diagnosis

○ *Tiny foci of involvement and clinical history help to differentiate from other entities with similar histologic changes* (Figs. 6.13 and 6.14)

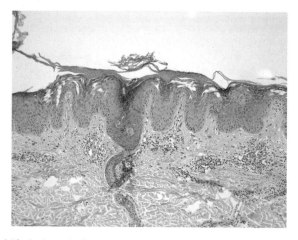

Fig. 6.13 In Grover's disease, many patterns of acantholysis may be seen, but they are small in scope. Original magnification 100×

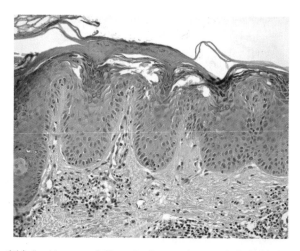

Fig. 6.14 In this case of Grover's disease, the acantholysis is superficial and resembles both Darier's disease and pemphigus foliaceus (in location). Original magnification 200×

- Warty dyskeratoma
  - Clinical
    - o Single lesion – usually on forehead, scalp of middle-aged to elderly patients
    - o Hyperkeratotic, may be cup shaped
    - o Rare cases described on oral mucosa and sun-protected regions
    - o *Clinical differential diagnosis usually includes basal cell carcinoma, seborrheic keratosis, and keratoacanthoma (not blistering disorders)*
  - Histologic
    - o Cup-shaped invagination at skin surface
    - o Central crater filled with orthokeratotic keratin
    - o Suprabasilar blister
    - o Abundant *corps ronds* and *grains*
    - o Pseudovillus formation
    - o *Striking resemblance to Darier's disease except for cup-shaped architecture*
    - o *Clinically distinct from Darier's disease* (Figs. 6.15, 6.16, and 6.17)

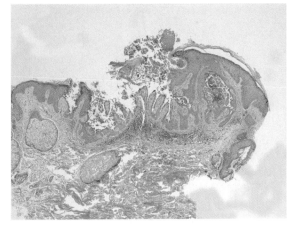

Fig. 6.15 Warty dyskeratoma is characterized by its cup-shaped invagination down from the skin surface. Original magnification 40×

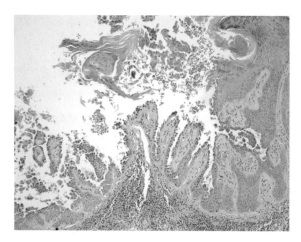

Fig. 6.16 There is a suprabasilar split similar to that seen in Darier's disease in warty dyskeratoma. Elongation of the rete ridges is also commonly seen. Original magnification 100×

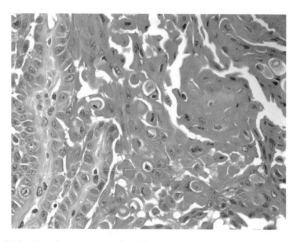

Fig. 6.17 Abundant *corps ronds* and *grains* are seen in warty dyskeratoma, identical to those seen in Darier's disease. Original magnification 400×

- Mid-epidermal blisters

  - Friction blisters

    o Mainly on soles from prolonged walking, or trauma-induced on palms
    o Necrosis of keratinocytes beneath granular layer
    o Degenerated keratinocytes on the floor of blister space
    o Minimal to no inflammation (Table 6.2)

Table 6.2   Blisters within the granular layer

Staphylococcal scalded skin syndrome
Pemphigus foliaceus/erythematosus

- Staphylococcal scalded skin syndrome (SSSS)

  - Clinical

    o Mainly in newborns and in children <5 years old
    o In adults, frequently associated with renal insufficiency
    o Diffuse erythema and fever
    o Large flaccid bullae and sheets of desquamating superficial epidermis
    o Mortality rate in children <4%, but >50% in adults

  - Histologic

    o Split is below or within the granular layer (very subtle)
    o Only histologic finding may be the loss of the stratum corneum that has separated in vivo or artifactually during processing
    o Rare acantholytic cells in granular layer
    o Virtually no inflammation
    o Gram stains are negative
    o *Differentiate from toxic epidermal necrolysis (TEN) by level of desquamation*

      TEN – separation below epidermis – full thickness sheet of necrotic epidermis
      SSSS – separation in granular layer – only a thin strip of necrotic epidermis (Fig. 6.18)

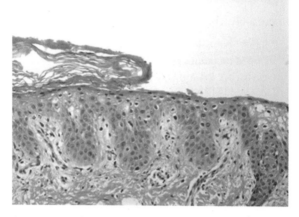

Fig. 6.18 A non-inflammatory blister is formed within and above the granular layer in *staphylococcal* scalded skin syndrome. Original magnification 200×

- Pathogenesis

  - Exfoliatin (exotoxin) produced by staphylococcal phage group II
  - Organisms not actually in skin
  - Newborn or damaged kidneys not capable of fully eliminating exfoliatin – systemic accumulation becomes toxic to epidermis

- Pemphigus foliaceus/erythematosus

  - Clinical

    - Flaccid bullae on erythematous base
    - Shallow erosions, gradually extend to cover much of body
    - May resemble an exfoliative dermatitis – blisters not apparent (+ Nikolsky sign)
    - No oral lesions
    - *Fogo selvagem* – disease endemic in parts of Brazil indistinguishable in all ways from pemphigus foliaceus

  - Histologic

    - Acantholysis and cleft formation within granular layer
    - May be only scant acantholytic cells

- o Grains (resembling Darier's disease) may be seen rarely
- o Eosinophilic spongiosis often present
- o Scattered eosinophils in dermis (Figs. 6.19 and 6.20)

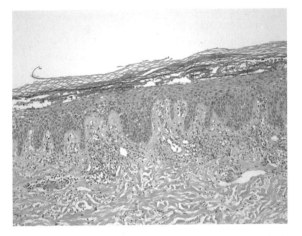

Fig. 6.19 Pemphigus foliaceus demonstrates a blister cavity within the granular layer. Scattered acantholytic cells are seen within the cavity. There may be occasional eosinophils. Original magnification 100×

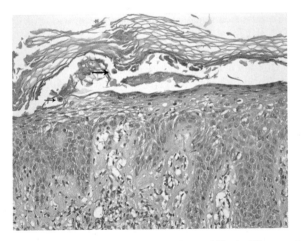

Fig. 6.20 Acantholytic cells (*arrows*) are present within the blister cavity in pemphigus foliaceus. Rare eosinophils are present within the papillary dermis in this case. Original magnification 200×

- Pathogenesis

  - Autoantibodies directed against desmoglein I
  - Chicken wire pattern of IgG and C3 around keratinocytes on direct immunofluorescence
  - Pemphigus erythematosus with same direct immunofluorescence staining pattern plus granular deposition of IgG and C3 along dermal epidermal junction

    Clinical relationship with lupus erythematosus remains unclear (Table 6.3)

Table 6.3   Subcorneal blisters

Erythema toxicum neonatorum
Subcorneal pustular dermatosis (Sneddon–Wilkinson)
Infantile acropustulosis
Transient neonatal pustular melanosis
Acute generalized exanthematous pustulosis
(Impetigo)
(Candidiasis)
(Miliaria crystallina)

- Erythema toxicum neonatorum

  - Clinical

    - Present at birth or shortly thereafter
    - Resembles acne vulgaris with facial papules and small pustules
    - Resolves rapidly without sequelae

  - Histologic

    - Subcorneal pustules with eosinophilic abscesses
    - Infiltrate in dermis of eosinophils and lymphocytes
    - No keratinocyte necrosis
    - In some cases, pustules appear to be at outflow tracts of acrosyringia
    - *Only subcorneal blistering process with eosinophils as predominant cell type* (Figs. 6.21 and 6.22)

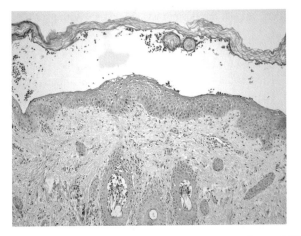

Fig. 6.21 Erythema toxicum neonatorum demonstrates a subcorneal blister filled with eosinophils. Original magnification 100×

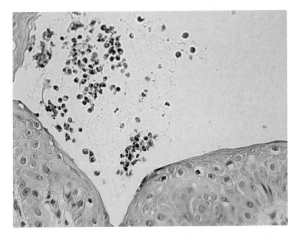

Fig. 6.22 In this case of erythema toxicum neonatorum, the blister cavity contains many eosinophils and neutrophils. Original magnification 400×

- Subcorneal pustular dermatosis (Sneddon–Wilkinson)
  - Clinical
    - Small, clustered vesicles on erythematous base
    - Blisters described as half-clear and half-filled with "pus"
    - Rarely associated with immunoglobulinopathies, pyoderma gangrenosum, and lymphoproliferative disorders
  - Histologic
    - Neutrophilic abscess high in epidermis/stratum corneum
    - Spongiosis in epidermis, especially around neutrophils
    - Mild lymphoid infiltrate in dermis with occasional neutrophils
    - *May be histologically indistinguishable from pustular psoriasis and acute generalized exanthematous pustulosis (AGEP)* (Fig. 6.23)

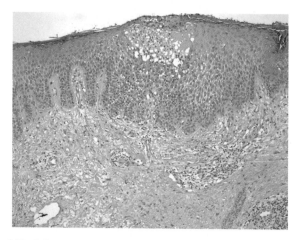

Fig. 6.23 Subcorneal pustular dermatosis (Sneddon–Wilkinson) demonstrates a subcorneal pustule filled with neutrophils. This may be difficult to distinguish from the changes seen in pustular psoriasis. Original magnification 100×

- Infantile acropustulosis

  - Clinical

    - o Intensely pruritic pustules on erythematous base on palms and soles of infants
    - o Evolving association with scabetic infestation in many cases

  - Histologic

    - o Acral skin with subcorneal neutrophilic pustules
    - o Mild accompanying spongiosis
    - o Rare eosinophils present but not the dominant cell type
    - o *Difficult to distinguish from pustular psoriasis or acute generalized exanthematous pustulosis (AGEP) without clinical history* (Fig. 6.24)

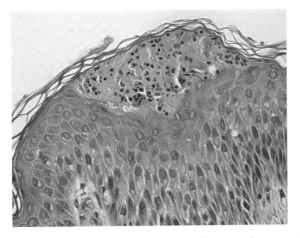

Fig. 6.24 Infantile acropustulosis is characterized by subcorneal neutrophilic blisters. There are no other distinguishing features other than history. Original magnification 400×

- Transient neonatal pustular melanosis

  - Clinical

    - Small vesicles and pustules evolve into hyperpigmented macules
    - Occurs exclusively in dark-skinned patients
    - Lesions resolve into hyperpigmented macules within 3 weeks to 3 months
    - Unassociated with systemic conditions

  - Histologic

    - Subcorneal pustules – predominantly neutrophilic
    - *Minority population of eosinophils present in some cases making distinction from erythema toxicum neonatorum difficult* (Fig. 6.25)

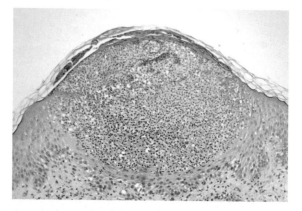

Fig. 6.25 Transient neonatal pustular melanosis is characterized by a subcorneal neutrophilic pustule on an acral site, usually in patients with darker skin colors. Original magnification 200×

- Acute generalized exanthematous pustulosis (AGEP)

  - Clinical

    - Diffuse macular eruption with pustules
    - Often abrupt onset within 2 weeks of initiating antibiotics

- o Usually associated with penicillins, cephalosporins
- o Resolves with cessation of drug therapy

- Histologic

  - o Neutrophilic abscess high in epidermis/stratum corneum
  - o Spongiosis in epidermis, especially around neutrophils
  - o Mild lymphoid infiltrate in dermis with occasional neutrophils
  - o Dermal eosinophils often present
  - o *May be histologically indistinguishable from pustular psoriasis and subcorneal pustular dermatosis* (Figs. 6.26 and 6.27)

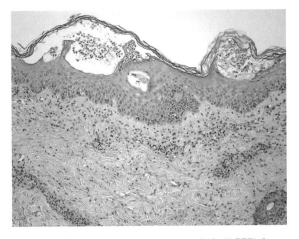

Fig. 6.26 Acute generalized exanthematous pustulosis (AGEP) demonstrates subcorneal neutrophilic pustules. In some cases, a dermal inflammatory infiltrate, often containing some neutrophils, is also present. Original magnification 100×

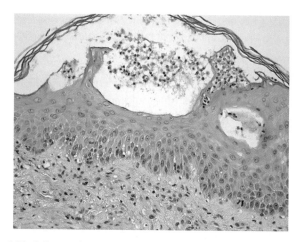

Fig. 6.27 Subcorneal neutrophilic pustules without bacteria are seen in AGEP. Scattered eosinophils are not unusual in this entity. Original magnification 200×

Chapter 7
Granulomatous Dermatitis

- Granulomatous dermatitis

  - Granulomas with acellular centers
  - Granulomas with cellular centers

    o Can be viable cells or necrotic cells (Table 7.1)

Table 7.1 Granulomas with acellular centers

Granuloma annulare
Annular elastolytic granuloma
Necrobiosis lipoidica
Rheumatoid nodule
Palisaded neutrophilic dermatosis of rheumatoid arthritis
Necrobiotic xanthogranuloma

- Granuloma annulare

  - Clinical

    o Small, firm, asymptomatic, pale red papules grouped in a circinate configuration
    o One to many lesions
    o Most common on hands and feet
    o Chronic, persistent, difficult to treat

B.R. Smoller, K.M. Hiatt, *Inflammatory Dermatoses: The Basics*,
DOI 10.1007/978-1-4419-6004-7_7,
© Springer Science+Business Media, LLC 2010

- ○ Disseminated variant associated with pregnancy, diabetes
- ○ Subcutaneous variant – children

- – Histologic

  - ○ Palisading variant

    Small foci of mucinous degeneration of collagen in superficial reticular dermis

    Often multiple foci in one punch biopsy specimen

    Palisade of histiocytes surrounding these foci

    Giant cells rare

    Lymphocytes, neutrophils (especially in early lesions), and rare eosinophils present

    Early lesions may have small foci that resemble mild LCV and demonstrate IgM and C3 in vessel walls (unusual) (Figs. 7.1, 7.2, and 7.3)

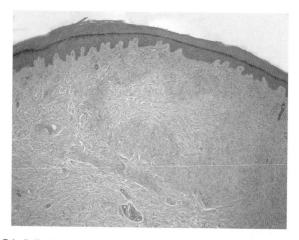

Fig. 7.1 Palisades of histiocytes surround areas of degenerating collagen in the superficial reticular dermis in granuloma annulare. Original magnification 40×

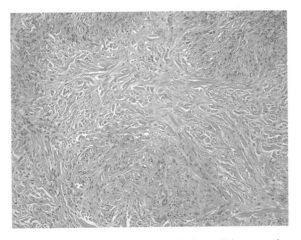

Fig. 7.2 The foci of degeneration are relatively small in comparison with other granulomatous processes in granuloma annulare. Original magnification 100×

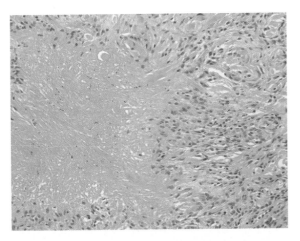

Fig. 7.3 Abundant mononuclear cells are present surrounding the areas of mucinous degeneration in granuloma annulare. Multinucleated giant cells are less common. Original magnification 400×

○ Non-palisading variant

  Diffuse foci of incomplete mucinous degeneration of
  collagen
  Histiocytes percolate individually between collagen bundles in linear arrangement
  Appearance at low power of a "busy dermis"
  *This variant may be difficult to distinguish from palisaded
  neutrophilic dermatosis associated with rheumatoid
  arthritis* (Figs. 7.4 and 7.5)

- Annular elastolytic granuloma

  – Clinical

    ○ Also known as actinic granuloma
    ○ May be variant of granuloma annulare occurring on sun-
      damaged skin, or a separate entity – controversial
    ○ Annular lesions, often on face, with raised borders,
      hypopigmented centers
    ○ May resolve without scarring after several years

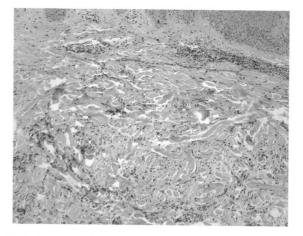

Fig. 7.4 In interstitial granuloma annulare, single histiocytes course through
collagen bundles diffusely throughout the superficial reticular dermis. Original
magnification 100×

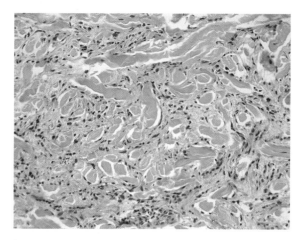

Fig. 7.5 Banal-appearing histiocytes are present between collagen bundles that show slight degenerative changes in non-palisading or "interstitial" granuloma annulare. Original magnification 200×

- – Histologic

    - o Small foci of complete elastolysis in superficial reticular dermis
    - o Foci surrounded by abundant histiocytes and giant cells, many containing elastotic material in cytoplasm
    - o Prominent asteroid bodies
    - o Elastic tissue stains highlight changes in elastic tissue (Figs. 7.6 and 7.7)

- • Necrobiosis lipoidica

    - – Clinical

        - o Irregular patches on shins with central atrophy and telangiectasia
        - o Yellow-brown in center, purple at periphery
        - o – Fifteen percent of lesions not on shins
        - o – Seventy-five percent in women
        - o – Sixty-seven percent with overt diabetes, virtually all with some glucose metabolism irregularity

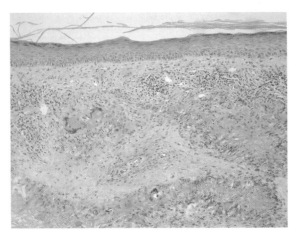

Fig. 7.6 Annular elastolytic granuloma is characterized by small foci of palisading histiocytes surrounding areas of elastolysis in the superficial reticular dermis. Multi-nucleated giant cells are usually abundant. Original magnification 100×

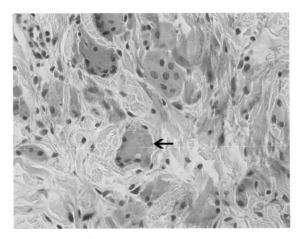

Fig. 7.7 Degenerating elastic tissue fibers are present within the cytoplasm of multinucleated giant cells (*arrow*) in annular elastolytic granuloma. This may be present on routine stains as shown here, or can be accentuated with a Verhoeff-Van Gieson stain for elastic tissue. Original magnification 200×

- Histologic

  o Large focus of necrobiosis in mid-reticular dermis
  o Foci of collagen degeneration may extend into subcutaneous fibrous septa
  o Pale-staining collagen surrounded by palisade of histiocytes, multinucleated giant cells
  o Dense lymphoplasmacellular infiltrate with germinal centers in some cases
  o Endothelial cell swelling
  o Vascular wall thickening (microangiopathy)
  o Histiocytes contain lipid in well-developed lesions (Figs. 7.8, 7.9, 7.10, 7.11, and 7.12)

- Rheumatoid nodule

  - Clinical

    o Subcutaneous, but may extend up into mid-reticular dermis

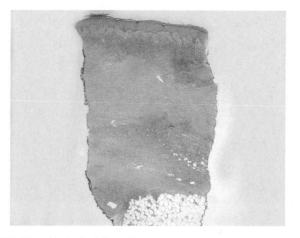

Fig. 7.8 Necrobiosis lipoidica (NL) demonstrates a stratified or "layered" appearance at low magnification with areas of cellularity alternating with paucicellular areas of pale-staining collagen. Original magnification 20×

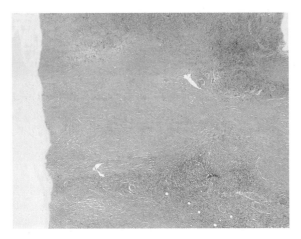

Fig. 7.9 The large areas of necrobiosis are pale staining and are surrounded by palisades of histiocytes and aggregates of lymphocytes in NL. Original magnification 40×

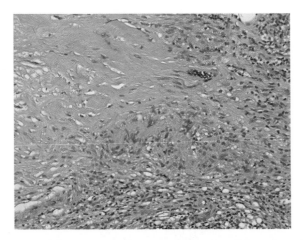

Fig. 7.10 Sarcoidal granulomas are seen in some cases of NL, as shown here, but may not be present in many cases. Original magnification 200×

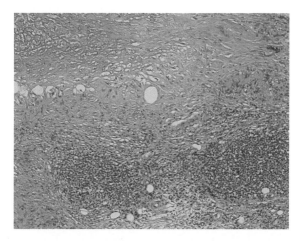

Fig. 7.11 In NL, there are dense aggregates of lymphocytes, often forming germinal centers. Occasional plasma cells may also be seen. Original magnification 100×

- o Most common in patients with rheumatoid arthritis, also rare in patients with SLE
- o Usually overlying joints on fingers
- o Children may demonstrate identical appearing nodules without other evidence of rheumatoid arthritis (likely subcutaneous granuloma annulare)

– Histologic

- o Sharply demarcated focus of fibrinoid degeneration of collagen in deep dermis/subcutis with "brick red" center
- o *Focus of altered dermis much larger than in GA and deeper than in necrobiosis lipoidica (in most cases)*
- o Focus surrounded by palisade of histiocytes, lymphocytes, and proliferation of blood vessels
- o Phosphotungstic acid hematoxylin (PTAH) stain demonstrates fibrin coating central focus of collagen

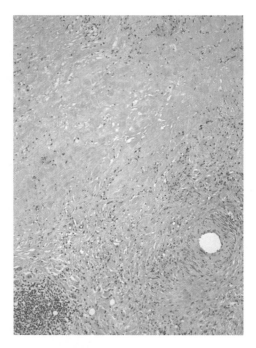

Fig. 7.12 Microangiopathy is seen in most cases of NL. Some authors believe vascular insufficiency to be causal in the development of these lesions. Original magnification 100×

- ○ *Histologically indistinguishable from subcutaneous GA in children – requires clinical correlation* (Figs. 7.13 and 7.14)

- Palisaded and neutrophilic dermatosis

  - Clinical

    - ○ Also known as interstitial granulomatous dermatitis with arthritis or rheumatoid papules
    - ○ Plaques, papules, or linear cords
    - ○ Lateral trunk is the most common area involved

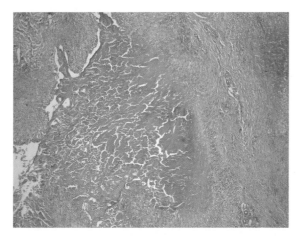

Fig. 7.13 Rheumatoid nodules are most commonly found in the deep reticular dermis. A large and bright red focus of collagen coated with fibrin is surrounded by a densely cellular palisade of histiocytes. Original magnification 40×

Fig. 7.14 The areas of paucicellularity in rheumatoid nodules are large and situated deep within the reticular dermis. Original magnification 100×

- o Associated with rheumatoid arthritis, lupus erythematosus, autoimmune diseases, hematologic malignancies

- – Histologic

  - o *Similar in appearance to granuloma annulare with more vascular involvement and less mucin*
  - o May be frank leukocytoclastic vasculitis (controversial)
  - o Often involves deeper dermis
  - o Extensive neutrophilic nuclear debris in most cases
  - o Some cases with C3, IgM, and fibrin in vessel walls on direct immunofluorescence (Figs. 7.15 and 7.16)

- • Necrobiotic xanthogranuloma (NXG)

  - – Clinical

    - o Large, indurated plaques with atrophy, telangiectasia, and ulceration on trunk
    - o Papules and nodules on face – especially peri-orbital

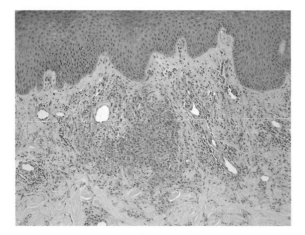

Fig. 7.15 In palisaded and neutrophilic dermatosis, foci resembling leukocytoclastic vasculitis are present with adjacent areas of single histiocytes percolating between collagen bundles. Original magnification 100×

Fig. 7.16 In other cases of palisaded and neutrophilic dermatosis, foci of mucinous degeneration are prominent, increasing the histologic similarity with granuloma annulare. However, there is usually more vascular involvement in these cases than is seen in granuloma annulare. Original magnification 100×

- o IgG monoclonal gammopathy (κ or λ light chains) in almost all cases
- o Scattered patients reported with associated multiple myeloma
– Histologic
  - o Large intersecting bands of granulomatous inflammation throughout dermis and into subcutis
  - o Bands of hyaline necrobiosis
  - o Foam cells, inflammatory cells (brisk), and abundant giant cells (Touton and foreign body types)
  - o Cholesterol clefts frequent
  - o Very extensive process throughout dermis
  - o *Much more florid change than in any of the previous entities described in this section* (Figs. 7.17, 7.18, and 7.19, Table 7.2)

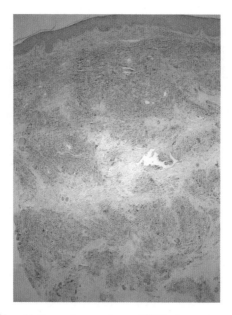

Fig. 7.17 Necrobiotic xanthogranuloma (NXG) demonstrates widespread degenerative change and granulomatous inflammation throughout the entire dermis. Original magnification 40×

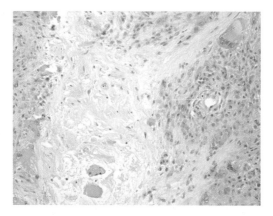

Fig. 7.18 Abundant large, multi-nucleated giant cells are present surrounding areas with complete dissolution of reticular dermal collagen in NXG. Original magnification 200×

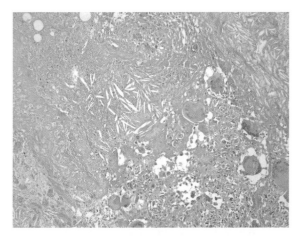

Fig. 7.19 Cholesterol clefts may be prominent in areas of collagenous degeneration in NXG and are usually surrounded by very large multi-nucleated giant cells. Original magnification 100×

Table 7.2   Granulomas with cellular centers

Sarcoidosis
Foreign body granulomas
Granulomatous rosacea
Infectious granulomas
Tuberculosis
Leprosy
(Cat-scratch disease)
(Sporotrichosis)
(Deep fungal infections)

- Sarcoidosis
    - Clinical
        ○ Transient form

            Associated with erythema nodosum, hilar adenopathy, fever, polyarthritis, iritis

            Persists only a few months, resolves without sequelae

        ○ Chronic persistent form

            25% with cutaneous lesions

- o Red-brown papules and plaques (lupus pernio)
- o Annular lesions
- o Occasionally lichenoid appearing
- o Rare subcutaneous nodules

  – Histologic

  - o Circumscribed granulomas with little to no necrosis
  - o Granulomas in papillary (characteristic) or reticular dermis and even into subcutis
  - o Giant cells not usually abundant
  - o Relatively scant rim of lymphocytes surrounding epithelioid cells
  - o Schaumann bodies – occur within old giant cells – laminated oval, blue-staining calcified bodies
  - o Asteroid bodies – also within giant cells – stain with phosphotungstic acid hematoxylin (PTAH), centers red-brown and periphery blue
  - o Neither is specific for sarcoidosis!
  - o *Diagnosis is one of exclusion and should be made only following the study of special stains for organisms and polarization examination and in conjunction with clinical presentation and laboratory data* (Figs. 7.20, 7.21, and 7.22)

- • Foreign body giant cell granulomas

  – Clinical

  - o Non-specific papule or nodule, often at the site of previous trauma
  - o Surrounding erythema related to associated inflammatory response

  – Histologic

  - o Irregular infiltrate of polymorphous inflammatory cells and scattered histiocytes and multinucleated giant cells

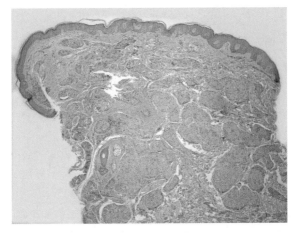

Fig. 7.20 Sharply demarcated granulomas are present at all levels of the dermis, with no predilection for cutaneous appendages in cutaneous sarcoidosis. Original magnification 40×

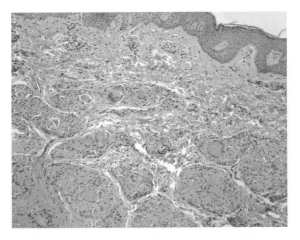

Fig. 7.21 Sarcoidal granulomas are comprised of histiocytes, scattered multi-nucleated cells, and only scant lymphocytes in most cases. Original magnification 100×

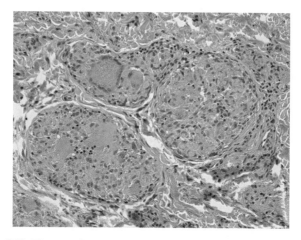

Fig. 7.22 The granulomas in sarcoidosis usually do not contain central caseation. They are sharply demarcated and have only scant surrounding inflammatory reaction. The centers of the granuloma are as cellular as are the peripheral zones unlike in granuloma annulare. Original magnification 200×

- o In some cases, polarization helps to reveal intracytoplasmic foreign material
- o Characteristic large, multinucleated giant cells
- o Character of associated inflammatory response is widely variable and depends upon host response and nature of foreign material (Figs. 7.23 and 7.24)

- Granulomatous (acne) rosacea

  - Clinical

    - o Lesions on center or lateral face
    - o Erythematous, telangiectatic patches, occasionally papular
    - o Papules are folliculocentric
    - o "Rhinophyma" is a glandular hyperplastic variant on face
    - o Eyelids involved in *lupus miliaris disseminatus faciei* variant

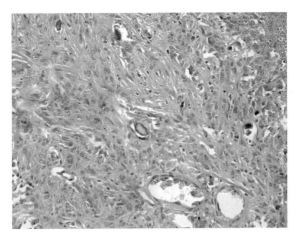

Fig. 7.23 Foreign material (*yellow*) is surrounded by an infiltrate of histiocytes in this foreign body giant cell reaction. Original magnification 200×

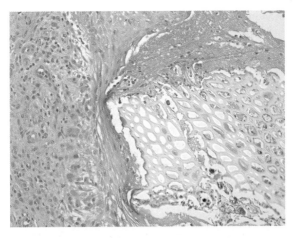

Fig. 7.24 A wood splinter engenders the same type of foreign body giant cell reaction with a palisade of histiocytes surrounding the foreign material. Original magnification 200×

- Histologic

    o Perivascular and perifollicular lymphoid infiltrates with follicular destruction
    o Spongiosis in infundibular region of hair follicles – most obvious in milder cases without granulomatous inflammation
    o Granulomatous response to destroyed follicles – keratin present in histiocytes
    o Caseation absent except in *lupus miliaris disseminatum faciei* variant
    o *Granulomas may be relatively "naked" and difficult to distinguish from sarcoidosis* (Figs. 7.25, 7.26, and 7.27)

- Cutaneous tuberculosis

    - Clinical variants involving skin

        o Primary
        o Miliary
        o Lupus vulgaris

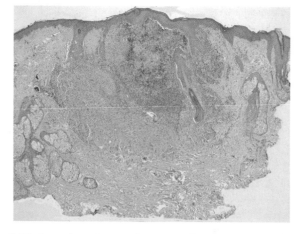

Fig. 7.25 Acne (granulomatous) rosacea demonstrates granulomatous inflammation around hair follicles. Original magnification 40×

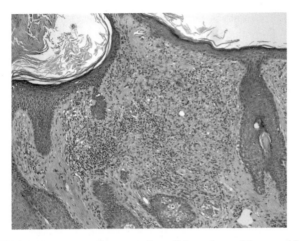

Fig. 7.26 In rosacea, granulomas may be well formed resembling sarcoidosis, but often have a more extensive accompanying lymphocytic response as is seen here. Original magnification 100×

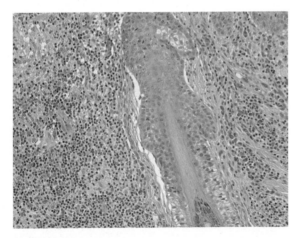

Fig. 7.27 The admixture of histiocytes and lymphocytes that characterizes most cases of rosacea is most prominent at the level of the follicular infundibulum. Original magnification 200×

- ○ Tuberculosis verrucosa cutis
- ○ Scrofuloderma
- ○ Tuberculosis cutis orificialis
- ○ Tuberculids

    Papulonecrotic tuberculid
    Lichen scrofulosorum

- Primary cutaneous tuberculosis

    - Vary rare
    - Acquired during mouth-to-mouth resuscitation, doing autopsy, tattooing
    - Many organisms present in areas of necrosis and in epithelioid cells
    - Later lesions may no longer demonstrate organisms (Figs. 7.28 and 7.29)

- Miliary tuberculosis

    - Rare, mainly in infants with disseminated tuberculosis

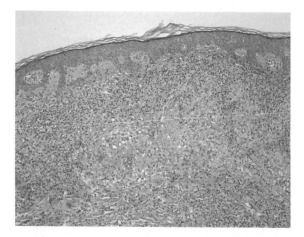

Fig. 7.28 Primary cutaneous tuberculosis is characterized by granulomas throughout the dermis. Unlike in sarcoidosis, there is usually a brisk accompanying lymphocytic host response. Original magnification 100×

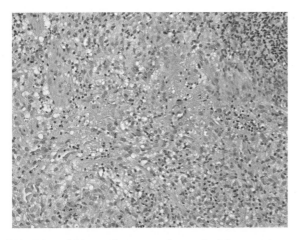

Fig. 7.29 Tuberculoid granulomas are characterized by central caseation (necrotic cells). Organisms are most commonly found on acid-fast stains (not shown here) at the peripheral edges of the necrotic areas. Original magnification 200×

- – All internal organs involved
- – PPD is negative due to anergy
- – Invariably fatal
- – Many bacteria seen within necrotic centers of granulomas

- Lupus vulgaris

  - – Secondary reactivation in previously infected patients
  - – Ninety percent on head and neck
  - – Red-brown patches with deep-seated nodules (apple jelly nodules)
  - – Tubercles seen in dermis, but caseation relatively slight
  - – Many histiocytes and giant cells but only rare organisms
  - – Epidermis – atrophic or hyperplastic
  - – Follicular destruction sometimes present (Figs. 7.30 and 7.31)

- Tuberculosis verrucosa cutis (verruca necrogenica)

  - – Exogenous infection in patients with high immunity

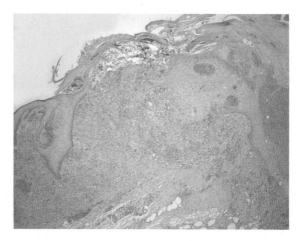

Fig. 7.30 Lupus vulgaris (cutaneous tuberculosis) is characterized by a granulomatous infiltrate underlying an acanthotic epidermis in which are frequently found neutrophilic abscesses. Original magnification 40×

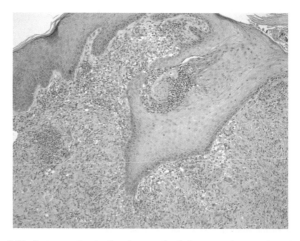

Fig. 7.31 Lupus vulgaris is characterized by granulomas that do not ordinarily demonstrate extensive caseation. Organisms are relatively difficult to find. Original magnification 100×

- Single verrucous lesion
- Organisms usually apparent on Ziehl-Neelsen acid-fast bacillus (AFB) test

- Scrofuloderma

  - Direct extension into skin from underlying bone or nodal infection
  - Abscesses seen superficially with caseating tuberculoid granulomas deeper in skin
  - Organisms usually abundant

- Tuberculosis cutis orificialis

  - Shallow ulcers with granulating base seen near mucosal orifices of patients with advanced internal disease
  - Many caseating granulomas with abundant organisms

- Tuberculids

  - Hypersensitivity reactions to organisms

    o No organisms actually present within these lesions
    o Caseating granulomas may be present in all clinical sub-types of tuberculid

- Leprosy

  - Classification

    o Polar tuberculoid
    o Borderline tuberculoid
    o Boderline
    o Indeterminate
    o Borderline lepromatous
    o Subpolar lepromatous
    o Polar lepromatous

- Leprosy

  - Clinical

- o Number of lesions and organisms increases with decreased immunity
- o Only polar forms are stable – others constantly shifting

- Leprosy

  - Tuberculoid

    - o Clinical

      One or few lesions
      Well-demarcated, asymmetric macules with raised borders
      Hypoesthetic
      Hypopigmented, loss of hair in lesions
      Impaired sweating
      Palpable superficial nerves near lesions

    - o Histology

      Epithelioid granulomas indistinguishable from sarcoidosis
      Granulomas may have oblong configuration due to surrounding nerves
      May be slight central necrosis in peri-neural regions
      Mild lymphocytic and plasma cellular infiltrate
      No Grenz zone
      Organisms rare to absent
      Presence of plasma cells, enlarged nerves, and oblong granulomas may help to distinguish from cutaneous sarcoidosis (Figs. 7.32 and 7.33)

- Leprosy

  - Lepromatous

    - o Clinical

      Initially with cutaneous and mucosal lesions
      Neural involvement later
      Numerous symmetrical macules – infiltrative and diffuse
      Leonine facies, loss of eyebrows and eyelashes
      Lesions not hypoesthetic

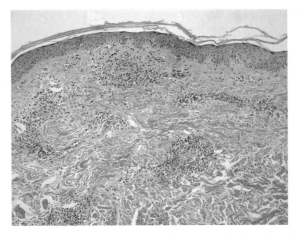

Fig. 7.32 Tuberculoid leprosy demonstrates scattered oblong granulomas surrounded by lymphocytes and occasional plasma cells. Original magnification 100×

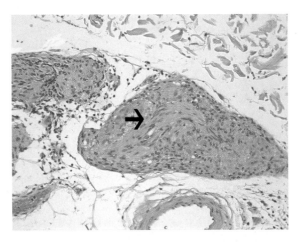

Fig. 7.33 In tuberculoid leprosy, well-formed granulomas are often found intimately surrounding enlarged cutaneous nerves (*arrow*). Original magnification 200×

   ◦ Histology

     Grenz zone
     Granulomatous infiltrate leads to destruction of appendages, extends into subcutis
     Virchow cells – macrophages distended with abundant organisms
     No granulomas
     Relatively scant lymphoid infiltrate
     Nerves less involved than with tuberculoid variant (Figs. 7.34, 7.35, and 7.36)

– Indeterminate

   ◦ Early in the course of disease
   ◦ Minimal inflammation
   ◦ Poor granuloma formation (Fig. 7.37)

● "Non-granulomatous" granulomas (misnomers) (Table 7.3)

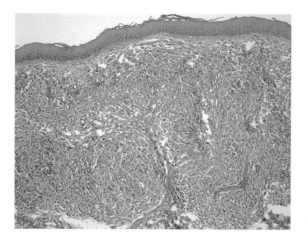

Fig. 7.34 Lepromatous leprosy demonstrates sheets of histiocytes diffusely throughout the dermis, underlying a *Grenz* zone. There is little accompanying lymphocytic response. Original magnification 100×

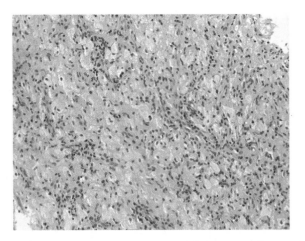

Fig. 7.35 In lepromatous leprosy, the sheets of histiocytes may be vacuolated and contain granular eosinophilic material (Virchow cells). These represent abundant intracytoplasmic organisms. Original magnification 200×

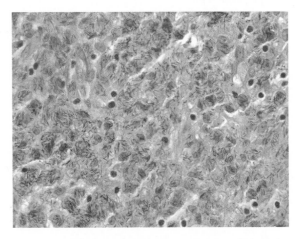

Fig. 7.36 A Fite stain demonstrates abundant organisms within histiocytes in this case of lepromatous leprosy. Original magnification 600×

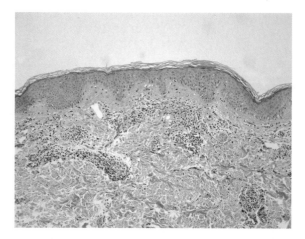

Fig. 7.37 Indeterminate leprosy may appear as a relatively mild superficial perivascular lymphocytic infiltrate with only rare histiocytes. It is quite difficult to make a histologic diagnosis at this point in the course of the disease. Original magnification 100×

Table 7.3   Non-granulomatous granulomas (misnomers)

Entity	Histologic pattern
Granuloma faciale	Resembles leukocytoclastic vasculitis
Eosinophilic granuloma	Langerhans cell histiocytosis
Lethal midline granuloma	T-cell lymphoma
Pyogenic granuloma	Lobular capillary hemangioma
Granuloma gluteale infantum	Spongiotic dermatitis (usually)

Chapter 8
Cutaneous Vasculitis

- Vasculitis

  - Definition

    o Inflammatory infiltrate leading to destruction of vascular walls
    o Histologic features required for diagnosis

      Transmural vascular inflammation
      Deposition of fibrin in vessel walls
      Evidence of endothelial cell damage
      Extravasation of erythrocytes

- Classification

  - Small vessel involvement
  - Medium-sized vessel involvement
  - Large vessel involvement - true large vessels are not present in skin

    o Arteries
    o Veins

  - Obstructive vasculopathies (not vasculitis)

- Additional Classification

  - Predominantly neutrophilic infiltrate
  - Predominantly lymphocytic infiltrate
  - Granulomatous infiltrate

B.R. Smoller, K.M. Hiatt, *Inflammatory Dermatoses: The Basics*,
DOI 10.1007/978-1-4419-6004-7_8,
© Springer Science+Business Media, LLC 2010

- Small vessel vasculitis

  - Neutrophil predominant

    o Leukocytoclastic vasculitis (LCV)

- Leukocytoclastic vasculitis

  - Neutrophilic vasculitis involving post-capillary venules in superficial vascular plexus
  - Most common type of cutaneous vasculitis
  - May be limited to skin or a manifestation of systemic disease
  - Often associated with infections, connective tissue diseases, drug exposure, malignancy – due to circulating immune complexes
  - Clinical

    o Most common on lower extremities but may generalize
    o Non-blanchable, purpuric papules
    o May ulcerate
    o Some lesions may appear urticarial or bullous

  - Raises a differential diagnosis

    o Henoch–Schönlein purpura
    o Drug reaction
    o Infectious etiology
    o Erythema elevatum diutinum
    o Granuloma faciale
    o Cryoglobulinemia (mixed type)
    o Connective tissue disease (systemic lupus erythematosus, rheumatoid arthritis)
    o Sometimes manifestation of polyarteritis, Wegener's granulomatosis, allergic granulomatosis

  - Histologic

    o Neutrophilic infiltrate invading venules of superficial vascular plexus
    o Vascular wall destruction, scattered thrombi
    o Karyorrhectic debris commonly seen
    o Extravasation of erythrocytes

- o May extend into deeper dermis
- o Presence of many eosinophils may suggest drug-induced vasculitis
- o Direct immunofluorescence demonstrates IgG, C3, and fibrin within and around affected dermal blood vessels
- o IgA and IgM less commonly present (Figs. 8.1, 8.2, and 8.3)

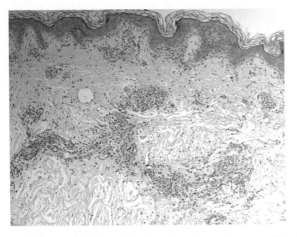

Fig. 8.1 Leukocytoclastic vasculitis shows a perivascular neutrophilic infiltrate on low power. Although the epidermis looks uninvolved in this case, there may also be, secondary to the vascular compromise, overlying epidermal changes of ischemia, including spongiosis, interface degeneration, epidermal necrosis, and bullae

- Henoch–Schönlein purpura

  – Clinical

    - o Usually in children
    - o Petechiae, ecchymoses, urticaria, bullae
    - o Arthralgias, abdominal pain, hematuria
    - o Usually lasts about 4 weeks, but 40% with recurrence (especially in adults)

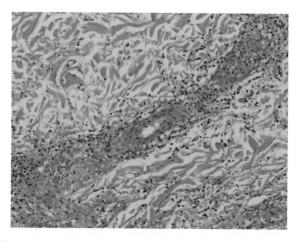

Fig. 8.2 In this case of leukocytoclastic vasculitis, fibrinoid necrosis of the vascular wall is extensive

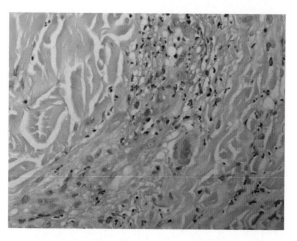

Fig. 8.3 Leukocytoclastic vasculitis shows reactive endothelium with plump endothelial cells, transmural migration of neutrophils, and fibrin thrombi, in addition to vascular wall necrosis

- Histologic

  o Leukocytoclastic vasculitis – no distinguishing features
  o Direct immunofluorescence demonstrates IgA and C3 deposition in vessel walls. As in all vasculopathies, perivascular fibrin will also be present

    Unaffected skin may demonstrate more intense immune depositions than markedly inflamed skin (Figs. 8.4, 8.5, and 8.6)

- Erythema elevatum diutinum

  - Clinical

    o Very rare
    o Red-purple papules and nodules symmetrically on extensors of extremities, elbows, and knees
    o Lesions become firm with age
    o Early lesions may be bullous

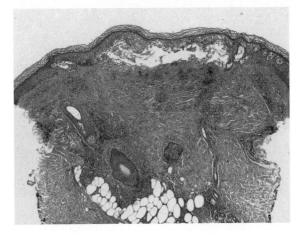

Fig. 8.4 Henoch–Schönlein purpura shows histologic features of leukocytoclastic vasculitis. This case also has epidermal necrosis and bullae, secondary to vascular compromise

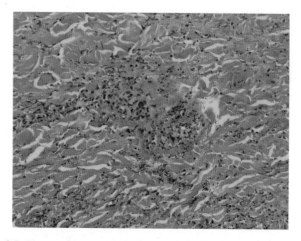

Fig. 8.5 The vascular assault in this case of Henoch–Schönlein purpura makes the vessels nearly unidentifiable. The focus of leukocytoclasis, neutrophils, and fibrin are the features that give a clue to the underlying process

Fig. 8.6 Direct immunofluorescence of Henoch–Schönlein purpura shows circulating IgA complexes deposited in the vascular walls (direct immunofluorescence, IgA)

       ○ Associated with monoclonal gammopathies (IgA, IgG) and mixed cryoglobulinemia

   – Histologic

       ○ *Early*: leukocytoclastic vasculitis
       ○ *Well-developed*: granulation tissue and fibrosis with persistent leukocytoclastic vasculitis
       ○ *Late*: cholesterol deposits within histiocytes and in surrounding dermis derived from long-standing, chronic cellular destruction (extracellular cholesterolosis)
       ○ Direct immunofluorescence – usually positive with immune complexes and C3 in vessel walls (Figs. 8.7 and 8.8)

• Granuloma faciale

   – Clinical

       ○ One or few slowly enlarging red-brown patches

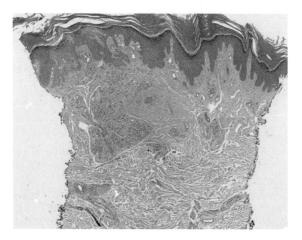

Fig. 8.7 This well-established case of erythema elevatum diutinum shows persistent neutrophilic vasculitis along with the stromal fibrosis associated with long-standing cases

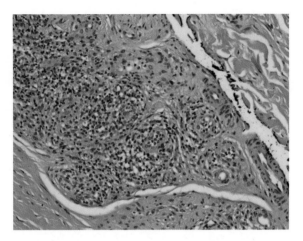

Fig. 8.8 This higher power image of late-stage erythema elevatum diutinum shows persistent vasculitis with a small neutrophilic infiltrate and perivascular granulomas and stromal fibrosis, consistent with a long-standing process

- o Almost always limited to face
- o Rare lesions on back, forearms

- – Histologic

  - o Misnomer – nothing granulomatous
  - o Dense infiltrate in upper half of dermis
  - o Prominent *Grenz* zone surrounding cutaneous appendages as well as along dermal–epidermal junction
  - o Leukocytoclastic vasculitis with abundant eosinophils, plasma cells, mast cells
  - o Extravasated erythrocytes
  - o Direct immunofluorescence – band-like deposits of IgG and C3 (also IgM, IgA) along dermal–epidermal junction and in vessel walls (Figs. 8.9 and 8.10)

- Cryoglobulinemia

  - – Only mixed type (associated with connective tissue diseases) demonstrates leukocytoclastic vasculitis
  - – Monoclonal types are non-inflammatory

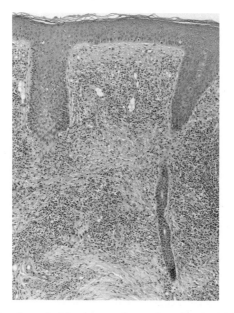

Fig. 8.9 Granuloma faciale shows a dense, dermal, mixed inflammatory infiltrate with an abundance of eosinophils. An uninvolved zone around the epidermis, the Grenz zone, is characteristic of granuloma faciale

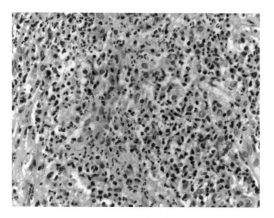

Fig. 8.10 The vascular inflammatory infiltrate in granuloma faciale is neutrophilic admixed with numerous eosinophils. Erythrocyte extravasation is also noted

- Histologically indistinguishable from other types of leuko-cytoclastic vasculitis

  o Very rarely can see crystalline-appearing material within vascular lumina

- Small vessel vasculitis

  - Lymphocyte predominant

    o Pityriasis lichenoides et varioliformis acuta (PLEVA)
    o (Rocky Mountain spotted fever – Volume II, Chapter 1)

- Pityriasis lichenoides et varioliformis acuta (PLEVA)

  - Clinical

    o Papules and nodules with ulceration and crust formation on trunk and extremities
    o Most common in young adults
    o Individual lesions last days to weeks, but eruption lasts weeks to months
    o Multiple lesions at various stages, simultaneously
    o Lesions heal with varioliform scars
    o Relatively asymptomatic
    o Debatable if this is truly a "vasculitis"
    o Relationship with T-cell lymphoma very controversial – weak at best

  - Histologic

    o Parakeratosis
    o Vacuolar degeneration of basal keratinocytes
    o Exocytosis of lymphocytes
    o Many necrotic keratinocytes
    o Superficial and deep perivascular lymphoid infiltrate with exocytosis
    o Lymphocytic "vasculitis" with extravasation of erythro-cytes
    o Eosinophils and plasma cells most unusual
    o Rare atypical lymphocytes may be present (Fig. 8.11)

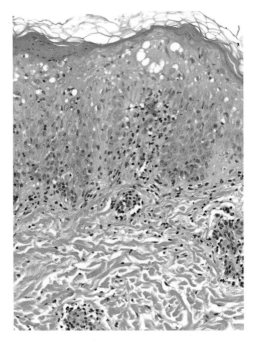

Fig. 8.11 This case of pityriasis lichenoides et varioliformis acuta shows spongiosis, exocytosis of lymphocytes, degeneration of the basal keratinocytes, keratinocyte necrosis, and parakeratosis. In the dermis, there is a moderate superficial and deep perivascular lymphocytic infiltrate

- Medium vessel vasculitis

  - Neutrophil predominant

    o Histologic changes are identical to those with small vessels, but involving larger vessels deeper within the dermis and subcutis
    o Usually systemic diseases

      Polyarteritis nodosa
      Superficial thrombophlebitis

- Polyarteritis nodosa

  - Benign cutaneous polyarteritis nodosa

- Microscopic polyarteritis nodosa
- Classic polyarteritis nodosa
- Benign cutaneous polyarteritis nodosa (BPAN)

  o Clinical

    Lesions predominantly in skin
    Usually nodose lesions, livedoid pattern much less common

- Microscopic polyarteritis nodosa (MPAN)

  o Clinical

    Associated with glomerulosclerosis
    Circulating antineutrophil cytoplasmic antibodies (P-ANCA)
    Patients usually with systemic symptoms
    More common in males

- Classic polyarteritis nodosa (CPAN)

  o Clinical

    Systemic disease involving medium-sized arteries
    Often associated with hepatitis B or other systemic antigenemias
    Livedo pattern very common, also purpuric lesions, erythema
    Nodose lesions are relatively less common

  o Histologic

    Neutrophilic vasculitis in all subtypes
    BPAN, medium-sized arteries in deep dermis/subcutis predominantly affected, superficial dermis rarely affected
    MPAN – usually involves only small capillaries, postcapillary venules, and arterioles, but not medium-sized vessels – strong histologic resemblance to leukocytoclastic vasculitis
    CPAN – superficial LCV and involvement of deeper vessels often seen

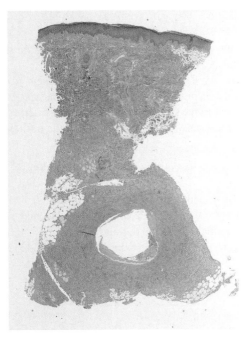

Fig. 8.12 Classic polyarteritis nodosa shows vasculitis of medium-sized vessels, which are located in the deep dermis and subcutaneous tissue

In general, histologic examination is not a reliable method for subtyping of polyarteritis nodosa – serologic studies and systemic workups are required to make this distinction (Fig. 8.12)

- Superficial thrombophlebitis
  - Clinical
    - o Pain, tenderness, erythema in linear distribution overlying superficial vein
    - o Associated with pro-thrombotic conditions including pregnancy, malignancy
    - o Mondor's disease – involves chest wall veins in patients with breast carcinoma

– Histologic

- ○ Neutrophilic infiltrate of medium-sized vein in subcutaneous fat
- ○ *May be difficult to distinguish arterial from venous involvement (and thus from polyarteritis nodosa)*
- ○ Elastic tissue stains may be helpful, but often elastic tissue enzymatically degraded by neutrophilic infiltrate

- Medium vessel vasculitis – granulomatous infiltrate

  - – Usually systemic vasculitides
  - – Involve medium or even large vessels, but may secondarily involve small vessels in dermis
  - – Characteristic infiltrate includes abundant histiocytes, giant cells, and polymorphous infiltrate (Fig. 8.13)
  - – Usually involves mainly arteries

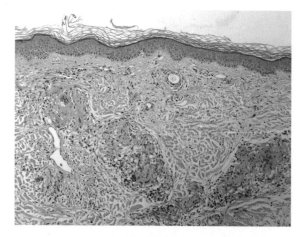

Fig. 8.13 Polyarteritis nodosa shows a perivascular granulomatous infiltrate. Extravasation of erythrocytes is seen in many cases. The overlying epidermis is not involved

- Granulomatous vasculitis

  – Wegener's granulomatosis
  – Allergic granulomatosis
  – Lymphomatoid granulomatosis (Volume IV)

- Wegener's granulomatosis

  – Clinical

    o Primarily involves lungs, upper respiratory tract, and kidneys
    o Fifty percent with cutaneous lesions
    o Papulonecrotic lesions with ulcers, petechiae, and ecchymoses

  – Histologic

    o Necrotic granulomatous areas with scattered epithelioid cells and foci of caseation
    o Necrotizing vasculitis involving arteries and veins (resembles leukocytoclastic vasculitis or can be granulomatous)
    o Any biopsy can demonstrate either or both of the above findings
    o Direct immunofluorescence demonstrates IgG and C3 within and around affected dermal blood vessels

- Allergic granulomatosis (Churg–Strauss)

  – Clinical

    o Sixty-seven percent of patients demonstrate cutaneous lesions
    o Papulonecrotic ulcers, ecchymoses, subcutaneous nodules

  – Histologic

    o Leukocytoclastic vasculitis
    o Similar mixed inflammatory infiltrate involving larger vessels deeper in dermis
    o Abundant eosinophils
    o "Flame figures" in interstitium

○ Extravascular granulomas very helpful if present
○ In some cases, histologically resembles polyarteritis nodosa (with abundant eosinophils) (Figs. 8.14 and 8.15)

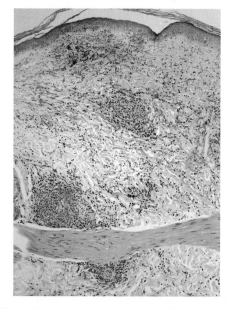

Fig. 8.14 Churg–Strauss shows a perivascular inflammatory infiltrate with numerous eosinophils

- Obstructive vasculopathies

  – Vascular destructive processes without inflammation (hence not "vasculitis")

    ○ Malignant atrophic papulosis (Degos disease)
    ○ Livedo vasculitis (atrophie blanche)
    ○ Disseminated intravascular coagulation
    ○ Coumarin-induced necrosis

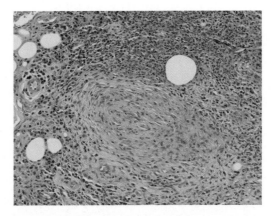

Fig. 8.15 Closer examination of the vessels in Churg–Strauss show perivascular granulomas and a dense eosinophilic infiltrate

- o Systemic emboli
- o Lupus anti-coagulant
- o Hyperfibrinogenemia
- o Monoclonal cryoglobulinemia

- – Histologic
  - o Similar changes in all obstructive vasculopathies
  - o Vascular occlusion by eosinophilic, acellular material
  - o Minimal to no inflammation surrounding affected vessels
  - o Affected vessels may be present at any levels of dermis but superficial vascular plexus most commonly affected
  - o Secondary necrosis of epidermis due to decreased blood flow may be seen in well-developed lesions
  - o *Clinical correlation and serologic studies are required to distinguish between obstructive vasculopathies* (Figs. 8.16 and 8.17)

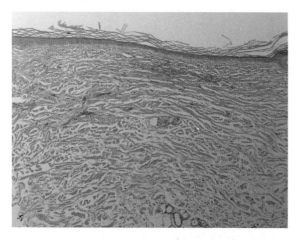

Fig. 8.16 As in other cases of obstructive vasculopathies, this case of monoclonal cryoglobulinemia shows a non-inflammatory vasculopathy with erythrocyte extravasation

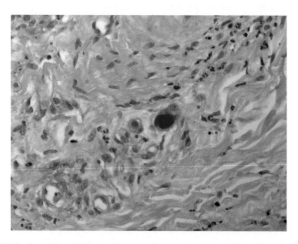

Fig. 8.17 Special staining in this case of monoclonal cryoglobulinemia shows PAS-positive, diastase-resistant material obstructing the lumen of vessels in the superficial dermis

Chapter 9
Alopecias

- Normal hair physiology

    - Anagen (active growth) – 89% of all hairs
    - Catagen (resting phase) – 1% of all hairs – for diagnostic purposes, not important – can be lumped with telogen as "non-anagen phase hairs"
    - Telogen (involuting phase) – 10% of all hairs

- Alopecias

    - Classification

        o Inflammatory

            Non-scarring
            Scarring

        o Non-inflammatory

- Inflammatory, non-scarring alopecias

    - Alopecia areata
    - Secondary syphilis
    - Follicular mucinosis (alopecia mucinosa)

- Alopecia areata

    - Clinical

        o Circumscribed patch of alopecia

B.R. Smoller, K.M. Hiatt, *Inflammatory Dermatoses: The Basics*, 179
DOI 10.1007/978-1-4419-6004-7_9,
© Springer Science+Business Media, LLC 2010

- ○ Exclamation point hairs
- ○ Preservation of follicular orifices in areas of alopecia
- ○ Minimal erythema
- ○ Can be diffuse – alopecia totalis or universalis
- ○ Associated with other autoimmune disorders
- ○ May also be autoimmune mediated
- ○ Prognosis – may resolve with therapy

- Histologic

  - ○ Sparse to moderate lymphohistiocytic infiltrate in the bulb of anagen and catagen hairs
  - ○ Increased numbers of catagen (early) or telogen (late) hairs
  - ○ Miniaturization of hair follicles (late) and slight fibrosis, but no scarring (Figs. 9.1 and 9.2)

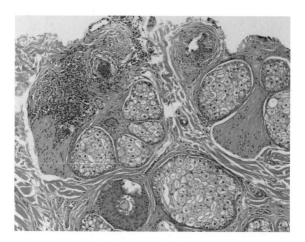

Fig. 9.1 Alopecia areata shows a moderate lymphohistiocytic infiltrate around the bulb of the hair as well as miniaturization of the hair follicle and increased telogen hairs

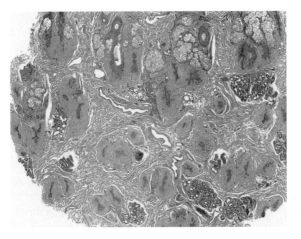

Fig. 9.2 In late-stage alopecia areata, there are numerous telogen follicles and no scarring

- Secondary syphilis

  - Clinical

    o Moth-eaten appearance to alopecia on scalp
    o Follicular ostia remain present – no scarring
    o Erythema and slight scale may be present
    o Associated with other cutaneous signs of secondary syphilis (Volume II, Chapter 2)

  - Histology

    o Perifollicular infiltrate of lymphocytes and plasma cells
    o Rare spirochetes may be seen on Warthin–Starry silver stain or anti-spirochetal antibodies
    o Changes are subtle
    o No scarring

- Follicular mucinosis

  - Clinical

    - o Primary (idiopathic) and secondary forms
    - o Follicular papules progress to boggy plaques
    - o Follicular ostia often patulous
    - o Lesions lack hair
    - o Primary type resolves in months to years
    - o Secondary type associated with mycosis fungoides (other lymphomas less commonly)
    - o Secondary type usually with more extensive lesions
    - o Secondary also reported with lupus erythematosus, verruca, angiolymphoid hyperplasia with eosinophilia
    - o Recent literature suggests that all forms of follicular mucinosis may be incipient mycosis fungoides – controversial!

  - Histologic

    - o Mucinous changes in outer root sheath of hair follicle and within sebaceous glands (earliest changes)
    - o Follicular epithelium undergoes reticular degeneration
    - o Cystic spaces filled with mucin (positive with colloidal iron or alcian blue at pH 4.5 or 2.5)
    - o Lymphohistiocytic and eosinophilic infiltrate
    - o In cases with clonality, the lymphocytes express CD3 and CD4 and are negative for CD8 and CD7.
    - o Gene cell rearrangement studies frequently indicated to exclude clonal T-cell population (Figs. 9.3, 9.4, 9.5, and 9.6)

- Inflammatory, scarring alopecias

  - Neutrophil predominant

    - o Folliculitis decalvans
    - o Acne conglobata, folliculitis abscedens, etc.

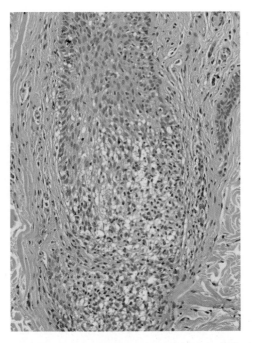

Fig. 9.3 Follicular mucinosis showing degeneration of the follicular epithelium with deposition of mucin and exocytosis of lymphocytes

- Folliculitis decalvans

  - Clinical

    o More common in males
    o Atrophic areas of alopecia with pustules at the peripheral margins
    o Can be painful, erythematous, and boggy

  - Histologic

    o Perifollicular neutrophilic infiltrate (early)
    o Later, plasma cells and lymphocytes predominate
    o Abscesses present may destroy follicular epithelium and result in granulomatous foci
    o Fibrosis and scarring common late (Figs. 9.7 and 9.8)

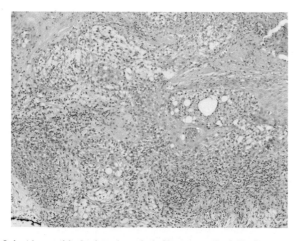

Fig. 9.4 Along with the lymphocytic infiltrate seen in follicular mucinosis, there is an associated eosinophilic infiltrate, which may be exuberant

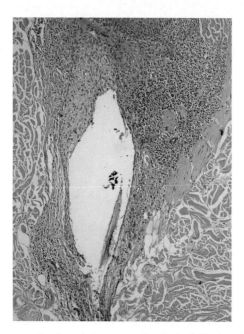

Fig. 9.5 Large pools of mucin can accumulate in the follicular epithelium in follicular mucinosis

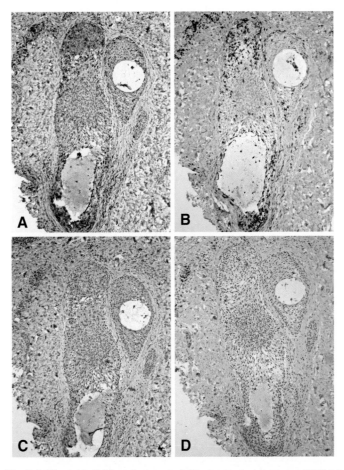

Fig. 9.6 The epithelial lymphocytes in follicular mucinosis express CD3 (**a**) and CD4 (**b**) and are negative for CD8 (**c**). With respect to CD3, there is loss of expression of CD7 (**d**)

Fig. 9.7 Folliculitis
decalvans demonstrates
a neutrophilic infiltrate
with scaring and
subsequent loss of
follicles

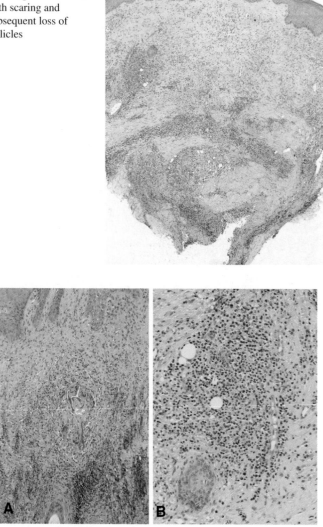

Fig. 9.8 The abscesses in folliculitis decalvans disrupt the follicular epithelium resulting in granulomatous foci (**a**). In this late-stage case, the infiltrate
has shifted to primarily lymphocytes and plasma cells (**b**)

- Inflammatory, scarring alopecias

  – Lymphocyte predominant

    o Lupus erythematosus (also Volume II, Chapter 2)
    o Lichen planopilaris
    o Pseudopelade of Brocq

- Lupus erythematosus (discoid)

  – Clinical

    o Scaly, erythematous, annular plaques without hair
    o Prominent follicular plugging
    o Often prominent involvement in external ear canals
    o Clinically, relatively non-inflammatory
    o Can occur in systemic LE or as isolated cutaneous eruption
    o Prognosis – mixed, some resolve without scarring, others with scarring

  – Histologic

    o Epidermal atrophy (late finding)
    o Orthokeratotic hyperkeratosis
    o Follicular plugging
    o Superficial and deep perivascular and peri-appendageal lymphoid infiltrate (peri-eccrine inflammation is very helpful diagnostically)
    o Interface dermatitis with basal vacuolization
    o Basement membrane thickening (often difficult to recognize)
    o Slight increase in dermal mucin
    o Increased non-anagen phase hairs
    o Scarring late
    o Direct immunofluorescence

      Granular deposition of C3 and immunoglobulins at DEJ IgM and IgA may also be present in same distribution (Figs. 9.9, 9.10, and 9.11)

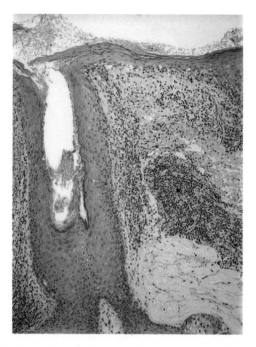

Fig. 9.9 In lupus alopecia, there is epidermal atrophy and exocytosis of lymphocytes into the epithelium (follicular and non-follicular). Epithelial basovacuolopathy and dyskeratosis are also present. A superficial and deep perivascular lymphoplasmacytic infiltrate is characteristic

- Lichen planopilaris
  - Clinical
    - Occurs on scalp or other hair-bearing areas
    - Resembles discoid lupus clinically
    - Hyperkeratotic papules surrounded by erythema
    - Occurs in older population and more in men
    - May co-exist with lichen planus (Graham–Little syndrome)
    - Prognosis – poor response to intralesional steroids

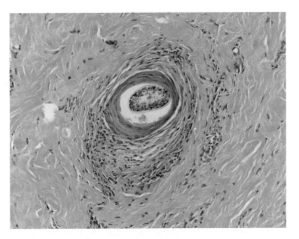

Fig. 9.10 Lupus alopecia results in the stromal fibrosis that is encasing this residual follicle

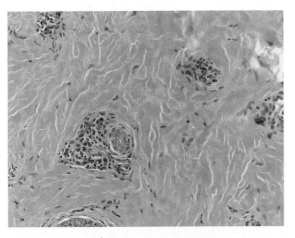

Fig. 9.11 Involvement of the eccrine apparatus, such as this eccrine duct, is helpful in differentiating lupus from lichen planopilaris alopecia

- Histologic

  - Lichenoid infiltrate of almost exclusively lymphocytes around hair follicles (resembles lichen planus)
  - Early – follicles and sebaceous glands disappear
  - Epidermis becomes atrophic later
  - Fibrosis replaces dermis
  - No peri-eccrine infiltrate (unlike lupus erythematosus) (Figs. 9.12 and 9.13)

- Pseudopelade of Brocq

  - Clinical

    - May not be a separate entity, but rather an end stage of all scarring alopecias
    - Irregularly defined, confluent patches of alopecia
    - Smooth atrophy, little inflammation
    - Persistence of few hairs within alopecic patch is characteristic

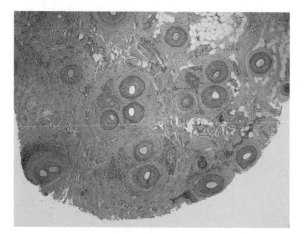

Fig. 9.12 Lichen planopilaris demonstrates perifollicular lymphocytic infiltrate with exocytosis into the epithelium. There is perifollicular fibrosis and follicular dropout and noted by follicular units with only one or two follicles

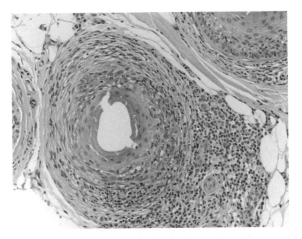

Fig. 9.13 This higher power image shows the extent of follicular epithelial involvement in lichen planopilaris. There is a moderate lymphocytic infiltrate with exocytosis into the follicular epithelium and dyskeratosis

- o Prognosis – dismal for hair re-growth due to obliteration of follicular epithelium
- – Histologic
  - o Sparse to moderate perifollicular lymphocytic infiltrate – especially in region of infundibulum
  - o Spares lower third of follicles (unlike lupus erythematosus and alopecia areata)
  - o Destroys follicles and sebaceous glands
  - o Fibrosis and loss of pilosebaceous units in end stage

- • Alternative classification of inflammatory alopecias
  - – Inflammation at the dermal–epidermal junction
    - o Lupus erythematosus
    - o Lichen planopilaris
  - – Inflammation at the follicular mid-portion
    - o Pseudopelade of Brocq

  - o Lichen planopilaris
  - o Folliculitis decalvans
  - o Acne vulgaris
  - o Secondary syphilis

  – Inflammation at the base of hair follicles

  - o Alopecia areata

- Non-inflammatory alopecias

  – All are non-scarring except if of long-standing duration at which point the hair loss may become irreversible

  - o Androgenetic alopecia
  - o Traction alopecia (trichotillomania)
  - o Effluvium (telogen or anagen)
  - o Trichodystrophies

- Androgenetic alopecia

  – Clinical

  - o "Male pattern" baldness
  - o Follicular orifices remain patent for long period of time
  - o Minimal associated erythema
  - o Autosomal dominant inheritance
  - o Can occur at any time post-puberty in men or women

  – Histologic

  - o Decreased numbers and size of hair follicles
  - o Increased telogen phase hairs
  - o Increased vellus hairs
  - o Minimal peri-infundibular lymphocytic infiltrate
  - o Increased size and number of sebaceous lobules
  - o No scarring
  - o Infundibular (as opposed to peri-bulbar) localization of lymphocytes helps to distinguish from alopecia areata (Figs. 9.14 and 9.15)

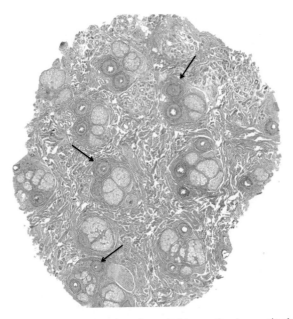

Fig. 9.14 This transverse section of a scalp biopsy of androgenetic alopecia shows 22 follicles, some of which are vellus hairs (*arrows*). Notably, there is no inflammation and there is a striking miniaturization of the hair follicles characterized by follicle diameters less than that of the sebaceous gland

- Traction alopecia
  - Clinical
    o Also known as trichotillomania
    o May be identical to "hot comb alopecia" and central centrifugal cicatricial alopecia (though the latter is often associated with scarring)
    o Physical disruption of hair by pulling, hot combs, and "corn rows"
    o Irregular pattern of alopecia without inflammation
    o Scarring develops only in long-standing cases

  - Histologic
    o Ectasia of follicular cavities with pigment casts
    o Trichomalacia: fragmented hair fibers often within dermis, outside of follicular epithelium

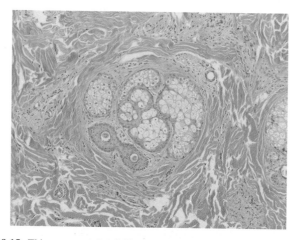

Fig. 9.15 This representative follicular unit in androgenetic alopecia shows loss of follicles and significant miniaturization of the hair shaft

- o Perifollicular hemorrhage
- o Epithelium separated consistently from sheaths
- o Granulomatous response with multi-nucleated giant cells in cases with extensive follicular disruption
- o Increased "non-anagen" hairs
- o Decreased total hair numbers
- o Occasional scarring if extensive and long-standing (Figs. 9.16, 9.17, and 9.18)

- Effluvium, telogen, and anagen

  - Clinical

    - o Increased shedding of hair
    - o Disruption of normal hair cycling
    - o In telogen effluvium, anagen hairs are prematurely shifted to telogen phase and extruded
    - o In anagen effluvium or anagen arrest, there is a loss of hairs from anagen phase
    - o Caused by metabolic alterations such as chemotherapy, pregnancy, stress, dietary imbalance
    - o Prognosis is excellent with reversal of underlying process

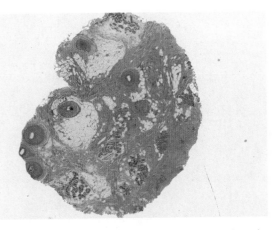

Fig. 9.16 This low-power image of a transverse section of traction alopecia shows hair follicle dropout, with only seven follicles in this 4-mm punch biopsy

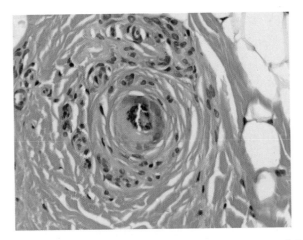

Fig. 9.17 This section of traction alopecia demonstrates an extruded hair shaft with associated multinucleate giant cell reaction

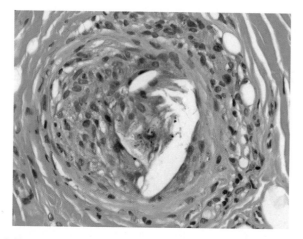

Fig. 9.18 Traction alopecia characteristically also has pigment casts and a granulomatous infiltrate

- Histologic

  ○ Anagen effluvium – normal anagen/telogen ratio

    Rarely see abnormally tapered hairs within follicles

  ○ Telogen effluvium – 25–30% of follicles shift to telogen phase with resulting loss of hair, increased catagen hairs; only rarely scarring (Figs. 9.19 and 9.20)

- Trichodystrophies

  – Structural abnormalities of hair shaft resulting in fragile hair
  – Acquired

    ○ Secondary to "permanents," bleaching, excessive sunlight, and, rarely, systemic diseases

  – Congenital

    ○ Rare, abnormalities in follicular keratinization; often associated with mental retardation, metabolic disorders, developmental anomalies

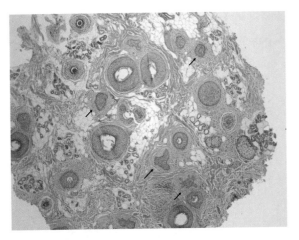

Fig. 9.19 Telogen effluvium in this transverse section of the deep dermis shows numerous telogen follicles (*arrows*), representing approximately 50% of the overall number of follicles

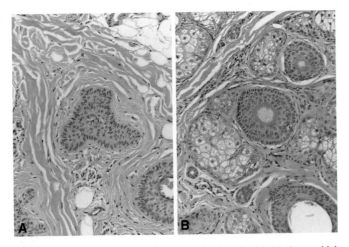

Fig. 9.20 Terminal catagen hair follicles in the deep dermis (**a**) show a thickened vitreous around the terminal germ unit with central pigmentation and pyknotic nuclei and in the mid dermis (**b**) the telogen hair has a serrated cornified layer interdigitating with the out root sheath

- Trichodystrophies

  - Acquired

    - Trichorrhexis nodosa
    - Trichomalacia
    - Spiral hair
    - Bayonet hairs
    - Pohl–Pinkus mark
    - Trichoptilosis
    - Trichoschisis
    - Trichoclasis
    - Pili bifurcati

- Trichodystrophies

  - Congenital

    - Monilethrix
    - Trichorrhexis invaginata
    - Trichorrhexis nodosa
    - Pili torti
    - Corkscrew hair
    - Woolly hair
    - Pili annulati
    - Pili bifurcati
    - Pili canaliculi
    - Trichothiodystrophy
    - Pili multigemini
    - Trichostasis spinulosa

  - Histologic

    - Diagnosis is not generally made on routine histologic sections, but rather on "hair mounts" taken from "hair pulls," often with the help of polarization microscopy (Figs. 9.21, 9.22, and 9.23)

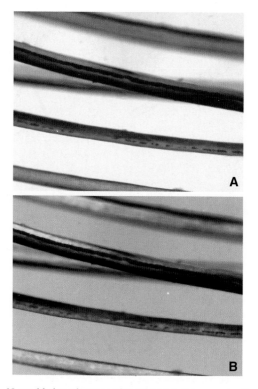

Fig. 9.21 Normal hair under transmitted light (**a**) shows a smooth outer cortex. Some shafts will have a central medullary canal. Under polarized light, normal hair shows (**b**) a variety of patterns, without a predominance of any particular pattern

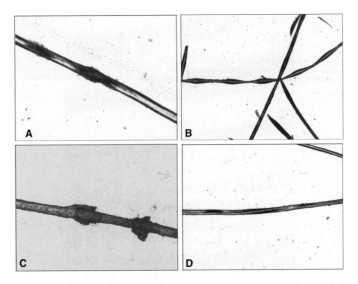

Fig. 9.22 Acquired and congenital trichodystrophies show characteristic hair shaft abnormalities that typically result is fragile hair. The defect in monilethrix (**a**) results in abnormal thinning of the hair shaft at regular intervals or "nodes." In trichorrhexis nodosa (**b**), there is loss of cuticular structure resulting in an easily traumatized hair shaft showing areas of fraying. Trichorrhexis invaginata (**c**) results when the proximal portion of the hair shaft is telescoped over the distal portion. In pili canaliculi et trianguli (**d**), under polarized light, a longitudinal groove is noted, which is formed from a keratinization defect resulting in a triangular prolife on cross section

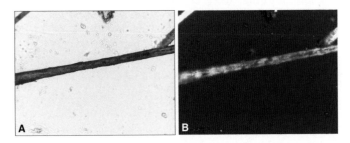

Fig. 9.23 Trichothiodystrophy, a defect in sulfur metabolism, results in hair that under transmitted light (**a**) have a regular appearance. However, under-polarized light (**b**) shows a very characteristic "tiger tail" banding pattern

Chapter 10
Panniculitis

- Panniculitis

  - Septal

    o Without vasculitis
    o With vasculitis

  - Lobular

    o Without vasculitis
    o With vasculitis

- Septal panniculitis without vasculitis

  - Erythema nodosum
  - Necrobiosis lipoidica (Volume II, Chapter 7)
  - Scleroderma
  - Subcutaneous granuloma annulare (Volume II, Chapter 7)
  - Nephrogenic systemic fibrosis

- Erythema nodosum

  - Clinical

    o Tender to painful erythematous nodules on lower extremities
    o Surface ulceration not present
    o Lesions last for months

B.R. Smoller, K.M. Hiatt, *Inflammatory Dermatoses: The Basics*,
DOI 10.1007/978-1-4419-6004-7_10,
© Springer Science+Business Media, LLC 2010

- o Chronic form – less common – lesions may last for years
- o Most common on young to middle-aged women
- o Associated with infections, oral contraception, inflammatory bowel disease, sarcoidosis, many other systemic antigenemias

- Histologic

  - o Septal inflammation with focal involvement of blood vessels (!), especially in very early lesions
  - o Lymphohistiocytic infiltrate with admixture of neutrophils and eosinophils
  - o Giant cells common in septa, often forming Miescher's radial granuloma
  - o Minimal fat necrosis present
  - o Later lesions with more septal fibrosis, less intense infiltrate (Figs. 10.1, 10.2, 10.3, and 10.4)

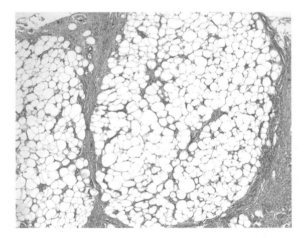

Fig. 10.1 In erythema nodosum (EN), the inflammatory infiltrate is largely confined to the fibrous septa between fat lobules, with only minimal extension into the periphery of the lobules. Original magnification 40×

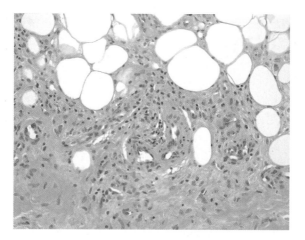

Fig. 10.2 In EN, along with lymphocytes, eosinophils and occasional giant cells may be seen within the septal infiltrate. Original magnification 200×

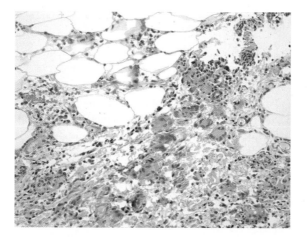

Fig. 10.3 Septal granulomas are present in some well-developed lesions of EN. Original magnification 200×

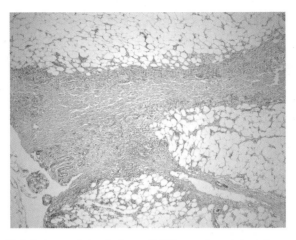

Fig. 10.4 Late, resolving lesions of EN are characterized by marked thickening and fibrosis of the septa between the fat lobules. Original magnification 40×

- Septal panniculitis with vasculitis

  - Small vessel involvement

    o Leukocytoclastic vasculitis (Volume II, Chapter 8)

  - Large vessel involvement

    o Polyarteritis nodosa (Volume II, Chapter 8)
    o Superficial migratory thrombophlebitis (Volume II, Chapter 8)

- Lobular panniculitis without vasculitis (Table 10.1)

- Lymphocyte predominant

  - Lupus profundus

    o Clinical

      Also known as lupus panniculitis
      Atrophic, depressed plaques on extremities

Table 10.1 Lymphocytic panniculitis without vasculitis

Lymphocyte predominant	Neutrophil predominant	Histiocyte predominant	Non-inflammatory
Lupus profundus	Pancreatic panniculitis	Subcutaneous fat necrosis of the newborn	Sclerema neonatorum
(Subcutaneous panniculitis-like T-cell lymphoma)	α-1-Anti-trypsin deficiency	Post-steroid panniculitis	
	(Infectious agents)	Factitial panniculitis	
	"Weber–Christian disease" (relapsing febrile nodular non-suppurative panniculitis)	(Sarcoidosis)	

May occur in patients with other stigmata of lupus erythematosus or as an isolated finding

Surface changes may or may not be present in overlying skin

○ Histologic

Mucoid degeneration and hyalinization of the periphery of lobules in subcutis – characteristic finding

Dense lymphoid and plasmacellular infiltrate, often with prominent germinal centers

"Rimming" of individual adipocytes by reactive T cells common (similar to finding in subcutaneous panniculitis-like T-cell lymphoma)

May be secondary vascular inflammation, but no definitive vasculitis (Figs. 10.5, 10.6, and 10.7)

- Neutrophil predominant
  - Pancreatic panniculitis

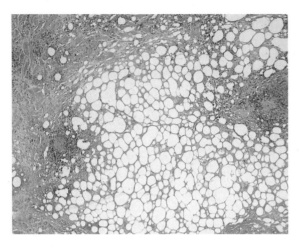

Fig. 10.5 A lymphoplasmacellular infiltrate at the periphery of fat lobules is characteristic of lupus profundus. Original magnification 40×

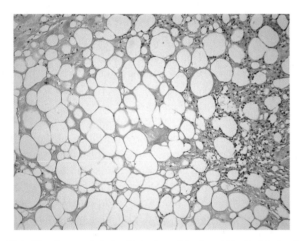

Fig. 10.6 The characteristic hyalinization of the fat within the lobules (especially at the periphery) is seen in this case of lupus profundus. Original magnification 100×

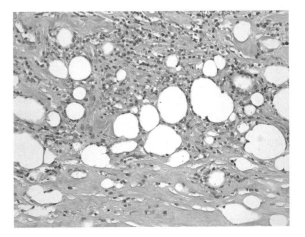

Fig. 10.7 Lymphocytes and plasma cells with occasional germinal center formation are seen at the periphery of fat lobules in lupus profundus. Original magnification 200×

o Clinical

Patients usually sick from systemic effects of pancreatitis

Areas of hemorrhagic discoloration, often on trunk and extremities

Ulceration with discharge of oily material through fistulae (necrotic fat lobules)

o Histologic

Multiple foci of diffuse fat necrosis across lobules

Presence of ghost cells (adipocytes) lacking nuclei

Calcium deposits frequent

Very brisk inflammatory infiltrate with abundant neutrophils, granulomatous foci secondary to fat necrosis (Figs. 10.8, 10.9, and 10.10)

- α-1-Anti-trypsin deficiency

  – Clinical

    o Patients often with long history of emphysema
    o Ulcerated nodules and plaques with oily discharge

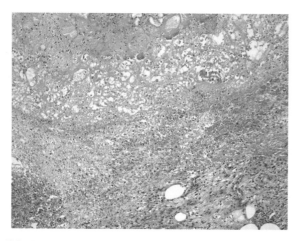

Fig. 10.8 Pancreatic panniculitis is characterized by abundant fat necrosis, hemorrhage, and an inflammatory response. Original magnification 100×

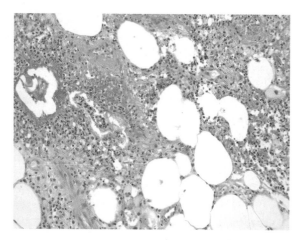

Fig. 10.9 A dense neutrophilic infiltrate within the fat lobules is characteristic of pancreatic panniculitis. Original magnification 200×

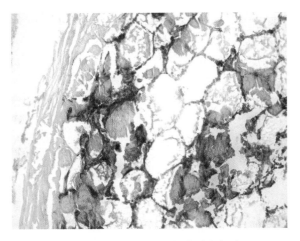

Fig. 10.10 Secondary calcification within the fat lobules is very common in pancreatic panniculitis. Original magnification 200×

- – Histologic
  - o Areas of normal, uninvolved fat adjacent to areas with widespread necrosis
  - o Extensive neutrophilic infiltrate throughout affected areas
  - o Hemorrhage diffusely
  - o Lymphocytes predominate at the periphery of affected areas
  - o No vasculitis (Figs. 10.11 and 10.12)

- • Weber–Christian disease
  - – Clinical
    - o Ill-defined entity that may not exist but may represent one of the many other types of panniculitis
    - o Crops of tender nodules associated with mild fever
    - o Mainly on lower extremities
    - o Lesions resolve with atrophic scarring
    - o Usually in middle-aged women
    - o Usually self-limited

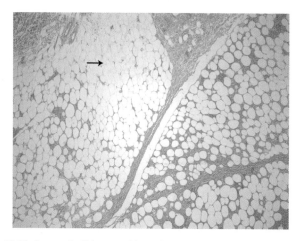

Fig. 10.11 In panniculitis caused by α-1-anti-trypsin deficiency, uninvolved zones of fat (*arrow*) are present adjacent to areas with widespread lobular fat necrosis. Original magnification 40×

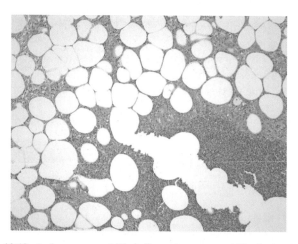

Fig. 10.12 A dense neutrophilic infiltrate is present within fat lobules in areas of necrosis in α-1-anti-trypsin deficiency-related panniculitis. Original magnification 100×

- Histologic

  o Three stages:

    Early – neutrophilic infiltrate of fat (short duration, rarely biopsied at this point)

    Middle – foamy macrophages associated with lymphocyte and plasma cells – diagnostic stage (if it exists)

    Late – fibroblasts predominate in healing phase (Figs. 10.13 and 10.14)

- Histiocyte predominant

  - Subcutaneous fat necrosis of the newborn

    o Clinical

      Nodules and plaques within days following birth

      Usually mild changes and patients are not sick, but rarely can be fatal

    o Histologic

      Fat necrosis within lobules

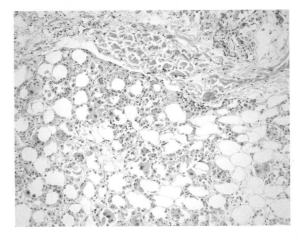

Fig. 10.13 Weber–Christian disease is likely not a discrete entity. In cases of subacute lobular panniculitis, a mixed infiltrate is seen within fat lobules and abundant lipid-laden histiocytes are seen secondary to fat necrosis. Original magnification 100×

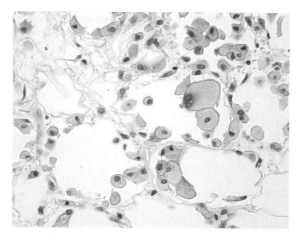

Fig. 10.14 Lipid-laden histiocytes are the predominant and most character-istic change in the so-called Weber–Christian disease. Original magnification 400×

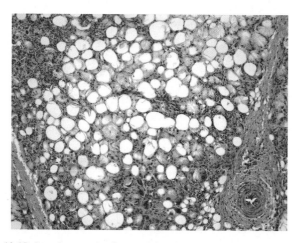

Fig. 10.15 In subcutaneous fat necrosis of the newborn, there is a dense infiltrate of lymphocytes and histiocytes within the fat lobules. Even at low magnification, cytoplasmic crystal formation is apparent within histiocytes. Original magnification 100×

Abundant mixed inflammatory infiltrate

Giant cells often with intracellular crystals due to degenerated fat (Figs. 10.15 and 10.16)

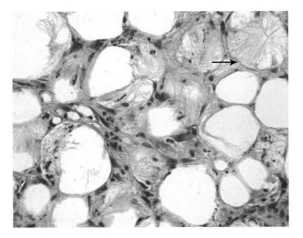

Fig. 10.16 At higher magnification, abundant crystal formation is seen within the cytoplasm of histiocytes in subcutaneous fat necrosis of the newborn. This is a very characteristic finding. Original magnification 400×

- Post-steroid panniculitis

  - Clinical

    o Occurs within a month after withdrawal from steroid therapy
    o More common in children

  - Histologic

    o Mixed, non-specific inflammatory infiltrate
    o Abundant neutrophils, histiocytes including multinucleated cells, lymphocytes
    o Spares vessels (unlike erythema induratum) (Fig. 10.17)

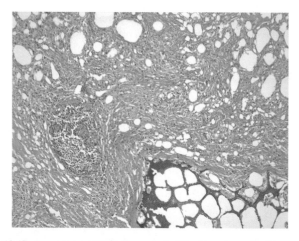

Fig. 10.17 In post-steroid injection panniculitis, there is a mixed inflammatory infiltrate predominantly within fat lobules. Blood vessels are spared and there is often fat necrosis as is seen in this example. Original magnification 100×

- Factitial panniculitis

  - Clinical

    o Characterized by clean, neat lines clinically and definitive, sharply demarcated patterns

  - Histologic

    o Non-specific
    o Mixed lymphocytic and neutrophilic infiltrate crosses lobules and septa
    o Variable numbers of giant cells are present depending upon degree of fat necrosis
    o Vessels are not involved
    o Polarization often identifies foreign material (Fig. 10.18)

- Non-inflammatory

  - Sclerema neonatorum

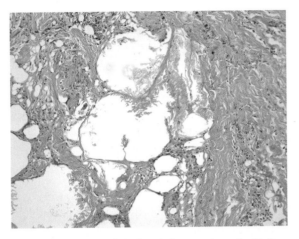

Fig. 10.18 In factitial panniculitis, there is fat necrosis, a mixed inflammatory infiltrate that may be present in lobules and in the septa. The blood vessels are spared. As is the case in this example, foreign material may be identified in some cases. Original magnification 100×

- o Clinical

    Associated with extreme prematurity
    Related to ratio of unsaturated to saturated fat and sensitivity to thermal factors (more saturated fatty acids – higher melting point, lower solidification point)
    Most affected neonates die in utero or shortly thereafter
    Diffuse, waxy firm change over entire skin
    Extremely rare

- o Histologic

    Enlarged adipocytes filled with needle-like clefts
    Usually no fat necrosis, inflammation, or calcium deposition (*death is too quick to allow for marked immune response*)

- Lobular panniculitis with vasculitis

  - Erythema induratum

- Erythema induratum
    - Clinical
        - Tender, deep-seated nodules, most commonly on calves
        - Lesions frequently ulcerate, heal with atrophic scars
        - Most common in colder months in middle-aged women
        - Association with tuberculosis continues to evolve

            Some DNA evidence for the presence of *Mycobacterium tuberculosis* in some cases

    - Histologic
        - Granulomatous tuberculoid infiltrate with caseation (present in about 50% of cases as a late finding)
        - Vasculitis of larger vessels common
        - Giant cells commonly seen
        - Plasma cells also present
        - Inflammation is predominantly lobular with ensuing fat necrosis
        - Stains for acid-fast bacilli almost always negative, despite polymerase chain reaction findings of DNA in some cases (Figs. 10.19, 10.20, and 10.21)

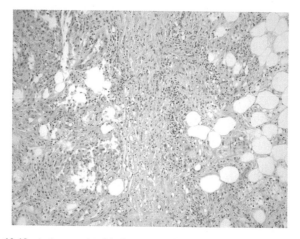

Fig. 10.19 A dense, mixed inflammatory infiltrate involving both the lobules (predominant) and the septa is present in erythema induratum. Original magnification 100×

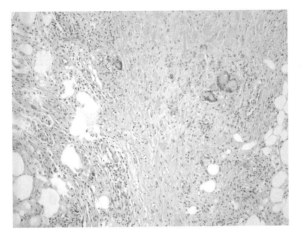

Fig. 10.20 Multinucleated giant cells and focal granuloma formation (even with caseation in some cases) are seen in erythema induratum. Original magnification 100×

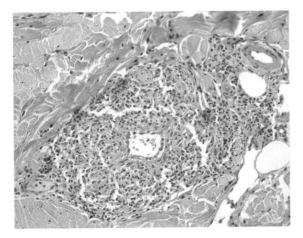

Fig. 10.21 The dense inflammatory infiltrate in erythema induratum may extend around and within vessel walls, and the presence of scattered neutrophils may raise the possibility of vasculitis in some cases. Original magnification 200×

Chapter 11
Histologic Mimics of Cutaneous Lymphoma

"Benign" infiltrates stimulating lymphoma

- T-cell mimics
- B-cell mimics

- Stimulators of T-cell lymphoma
    - Lymphomatoid papulosis
    - Actinic reticuloid (chronic persistent light reaction)
    - Anticonvulsant hypersensitivity reaction
    - Gianotti–Crosti syndrome (papular acral dermatitis of childhood) (Volume II, Chapter 3)
    - Cyclosporine-induced hypersensitivity

- Lymphomatoid papulosis
    - Clinical features
        - Usually affects young to middle-aged adults
        - Waxing and waning papules and nodules on trunk and extremities
        - Each lesion lasts weeks, but disease persists for months to years
        - Despite appearance, relatively asymptomatic

B.R. Smoller, K.M. Hiatt, *Inflammatory Dermatoses: The Basics*,
DOI 10.1007/978-1-4419-6004-7_11,
© Springer Science+Business Media, LLC 2010

- Histologic features
  - o Dense, "wedge-shaped" superficial and deep dermal infiltrate
  - o Exocytosis present in most (but not all) cases
  - o Predominantly lymphocytic infiltrate with scattered eosinophils
  - o Perivascular neutrophils frequently present – may resemble leukocytoclastic vasculitis
  - o Diagnostic cells are large, atypical lymphocytes, apparent at lower magnification

    "Type A" – resembles Reed–Sternberg cells
    "Type B" – resembles mycosis fungoides cells
    "Type C" – resembles Reed–Sternberg cells

  - o Can see both types of cells in any given lesion or in multiple simultaneous lesions from same patients
- Immunohistochemistry
  - o All are CD3$^+$ infiltrates
  - o CD4$^+$ cells constitute majority of infiltrating cells, including the large, atypical ones
  - o CD30 is expressed variably by the atypical cells depending upon the subtype

    "Type A" – most commonly associated with progression to lymphoma – about 20–30% of dermal lymphocytes express CD30
    "Type B" – variable expression of CD30
    "Type C" – most recently described – *histologically indistinguishable from large cell anaplastic lymphoma (>75% of cells express CD30)*

- Molecular features
  - o T-cell gene rearrangements are found in a significant minority of cases
  - o No relationship between detection of clonality and progression to lymphoma (yet discovered)
- Relationship to lymphoma
  - o Fifteen to twenty percent of patients with LyP will develop lymphoma at some point in their lives

- o Lymphoma may precede, follow, or occur simultaneously with the onset of lymphomatoid papulosis
- o Mycosis fungoides, Hodgkin's disease, and large cell anaplastic lymphoma are most common types associated

- CD30⁺ T-cell lymphoproliferative disorders

- o Spectrum of lymphomatoid papulosis and anaplastic large cell lymphoma

  In lymphomatoid papulosis a majority of the cells are reactive T cells surrounding a minority population of neoplastic T cells that express CD30

  Anaplastic large cell lymphoma has the opposite, i.e., the majority of cells are neoplastic cells that express CD30 and a minority of the population is reactive T cells

  New WHO guidelines views these entities as a spectrum of diseases (Figs. 11.1, 11.2, 11.3, 11.4, 11.5, 11.6, and 11.7)

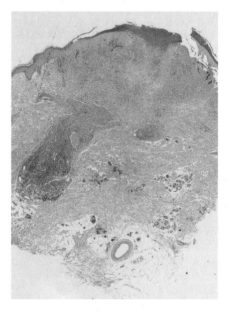

Fig. 11.1 Lower power image of lymphomatoid papulosis shows a dense, wedge-shaped inflammatory infiltrate

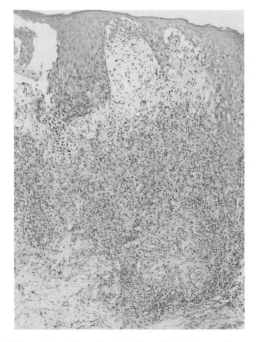

Fig. 11.2 This section of lymphomatoid papulosis shows a dense perivascular and interstitial infiltrate with prominent papillary dermal edema. There is exocytosis into the overlying epidermis

- Chronic actinic dermatosis (actinic reticuloid)

  - Clinical features

    - More common in adults
    - Begins as erythematous patches on sun-exposed areas
    - Eventually progresses to plaques and may generalize to involve sun-protected regions
    - Pruritus is common
    - Usually abates with sun avoidance

  - Histologic features

    - Epidermis usually with mild psoriasiform hyperplasia

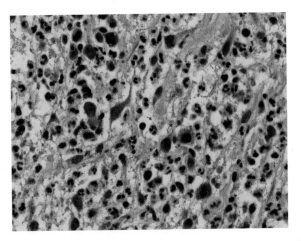

Fig. 11.3 The infiltrate in lymphomatoid papulosis has cells with striking cytologic atypia and may be florid as in this case

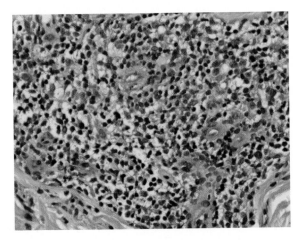

Fig. 11.4 In comparison to Fig. 11.3, the atypical cells in this case of lymphomatoid papulosis are not as abundant

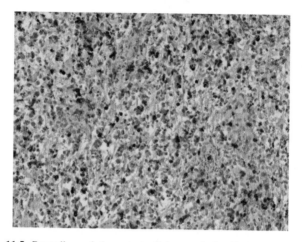

Fig. 11.5 Regardless of the extent of the atypical cells, the infiltrate in lymphomatoid papulosis is predominantly CD3$^+$ lymphocytes

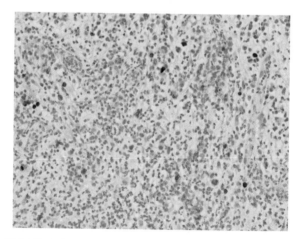

Fig. 11.6 The infiltrate in lymphomatoid papulosis has only a few CD79a-expressing cells

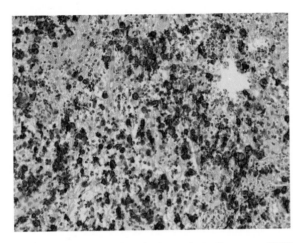

Fig. 11.7 In lymphomatoid papulosis, the atypical cells express CD30

- o Dense band-like infiltrate of lymphocytes within papillary dermis extending into epidermis

  Not lichenoid – does not obscure dermal–epidermal junction

- o Minimal accompanying spongiosis
- o Fibrosis in papillary dermis in long-standing lesions
- o Lymphocyte atypia variable
- o Minimal eosinophils or plasma cells

- – Immunologic features

  - o Infiltrating lymphocytes are mostly CD8$^+$, CD3$^+$, CD4$^-$ cytotoxic/suppressor T cells
  - o CD30 is negative

- – Molecular features

  - o Clonal T-cell gene rearrangements have not been described in chronic actinic dermatosis (Figs. 11.8 and 11.9)

- • Anticonvulsant-induced pseudolymphoma

  - – Clinical features

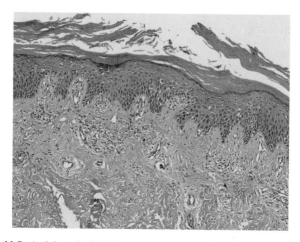

Fig. 11.8 Actinic reticuloid shows an acanthotic epidermis with an epidermotropic infiltrate

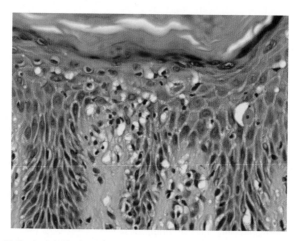

Fig. 11.9 Actinic reticuloid demonstrates an epidermotropic lymphocytic infiltrate with minimal accompanying spongiosis. There is mild atypia in the lymphocytes

- o Uncommon – occurs in <1% of those taking medications
- o Usually reversible with cessation of therapy
- o In florid cases, causes erythroderma resembling Sézary syndrome
- o Patients are clinically ill and present with hepatosplenomegaly, lymphadenopathy, fever, arthralgias, malaise
- o Elevated liver function tests

- Histologic features

  - o No characteristic changes in epidermis
  - o Dense infiltrate of lymphocytes within papillary dermis, occasionally extending deeper into reticular dermis
  - o Hyperconvolution and hyperchromasia of lymphocytes common
  - o Epidermotropism often present and may occur in the absence of significant spongiosis
  - o Pautrier's microabscesses in some cases
  - o Eosinophils present in most cases
  - o Lymph node germinal centers replaced with immunoblasts and "Sézary" cells

- Immunologic features

  - o Predominance of CD4$^+$ lymphocytes
  - o Minority of cells are CD8$^+$ T cells; B cells are rare
  - o CD30 is usually negative

- Association with lymphoma

  - o In most patients, eruption resolves quickly with cessation of drug
  - o In very rare patients, reports of progression to lymphoma
  - o Slight increase in lifetime risk of developing lymphoma for patients taking phenytoin (Figs. 11.10, 11.11, and 11.12)

- GLEEVEC-induced mycosis fungoides-like changes

  - Clinical features

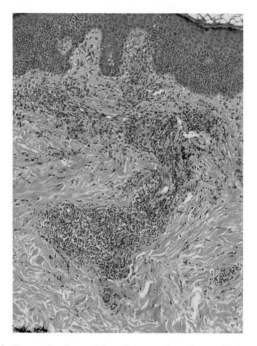

Fig. 11.10 Drug-related pseudolymphoma, or lymphomatoid drug eruption, on low power shows a dense dermal infiltrate without epidermotropism

- o Macular, erythematous, pruritic, diffuse eruption
- o Clinical differential diagnosis includes drug reaction vs. viral exanthem

– Histologic features

- o Superficial and mid-dermal infiltrate of lymphocytes
- o Epidermotropism of large lymphocytes with scattered Pautrier-like microabscesses and minimal associated spongiosis
- o Scattered eosinophils
- o No follicular mucinosis

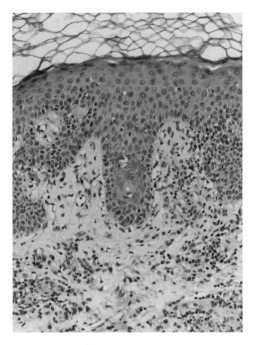

Fig. 11.11 This higher power image of lymphomatoid drug eruption shows a moderately dense infiltrate in the papillary dermis without significant epidermotropism. There is no associated epidermal change

- Immunologic features
    - Eighty percent of inflammatory cells express CD3
    - Equal numbers of CD4$^+$ and CD8$^+$ cells in dermis – *good discriminator from mycosis fungoides*
- Gianotti–Crosti syndrome (also see Volume II, Chapter 3)
    - Clinical
        - Also known as papular acrodermatitis of childhood
        - Originally described as representing primary infection with hepatitis B acquired through the skin or mucous membranes (especially ayw subtype)

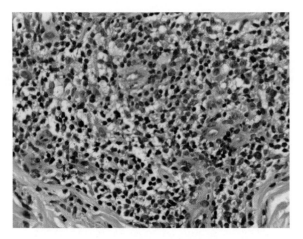

Fig. 11.12 A close inspection of lymphomatoid drug eruption shows a mixed mononuclear cell infiltrate with mild to moderate nuclear atypia, characterized by slightly enlarged, hyperchromatic nuclei with some nuclear contour irregularities

- o Now also associated with CMV, EBV, and coxsackie B viral infections
- o Non-pruritic, papular eruption on face, buttock, and extremities of children
- o Lesions persist up to 3 weeks
- o Lymphadenopathy

  – Histology

- o Moderately intense perivascular lymphohistiocytic infiltrate in upper dermis
- o Focal spongiosis, parakeratosis, and exocytosis of lymphocytes
- o Can see Pautrier-like microabscesses and mild–moderate cytologic atypia of lymphocytes

- Stimulators of B-cell lymphoma
  - Cutaneous lymphoid hyperplasia
  - Cutaneous lymphadenoma
  - Jessner lymphocytic infiltrate

- Cutaneous lymphoid hyperplasia

  - Clinical

    o Also known as pseudolymphoma, lymphocytoma cutis, lymphadenosis benigna cutis
    o Red–violaceous, tender nodules – can become quite large
    o Can be solitary or multiple, most common on face

  - Histology

    o Dense inflammatory infiltrate in dermis
    o Separated from epidermis by Grenz zone
    o May extend into subcutaneous fat
    o Usually small and large lymphocytes – often follicular architecture
    o Tingible body macrophages helpful in making diagnosis
    o May see reactive atypia, especially in long-standing lesions
    o Lymphocyte mitoses common
    o Presence of eosinophils and plasma cells is helpful in infiltrates with this architectural pattern

  - Immunophenotypic analysis

    o Nodules of B lymphocytes (express CD20, CD79a, CD21) with surrounding T cells (express CD3, CD4, CD8)
    o Majority of B cells express kappa light chains
    o Majority of T cells are CD4$^+$
    o Readily apparent CD68$^+$ histiocytes present throughout inflammatory infiltrate

  - Prognosis

    o Rare cases have been reported to undergo transformation to lymphoma
    o Retrospective study of tissue throughout course shows evolution of gene rearrangement and immunophenotyping patterns
    o Vast majority of cases resolve spontaneously or with minimal treatment

- Pathogenesis

    o Non-specific response to chronic antigen stimulation
    o May occur with no underlying etiology
    o Most commonly related to arthropod bites, ruptured hair
       follicles, persistent nodular scabetic reactions
    o *Easy to diagnose if identifying features such as punctum,
       keratin, or organisms are present* (Figs. 11.13, 11.14, and
       11.15)

- Cutaneous lymphadenoma

    - Clinical

        o Solitary, skin-colored nodules on scalp and face of
           middle-aged to elderly patients
        o Asymptomatic, slow growing
        o Non-descript

    - Histology

        o Obscure nests of epithelial cells not attached to overlying
           epidermis coursing throughout dermis

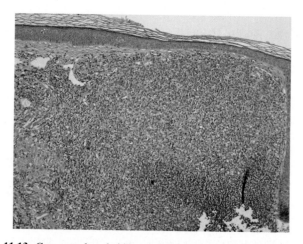

Fig. 11.13 Cutaneous lymphoid hyperplasia shows a dense dermal infiltrate,
typically nodular as seen in this image, with a Grenz zone

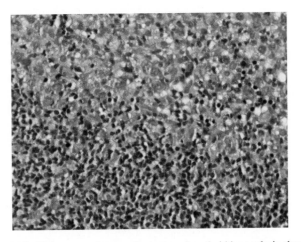

Fig. 11.14 Higher power image of cutaneous lymphoid hyperplasia shows a mixed infiltrate with foci resembling reactive follicles with germinal centers and tingible body macrophages

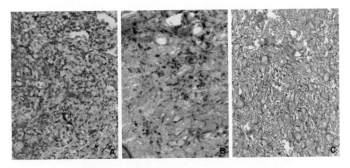

Fig. 11.15 Immunohistochemical staining of the infiltrate in cutaneous lymphoid hyperplasia reveals a mixed T-cell (**a**, CD3$^+$), B-cell (**b**, CD79a$^+$), and macrophage (**c**, CD68$^+$) infiltrate

- o Dense, diffuse lymphohistiocytic infiltrate largely obscuring epithelial proliferation
- o Spongiosis present within the nests of epithelial tumor cells
- o Epithelial component may be benign or malignant (lymphoepithelioma) and may show appendageal differentiation

- Prognosis

    ○ Depends upon cytologic features of epithelial component
    ○ Probably represents an appendage tumor (or more than one) with a massive immunologic response (Figs. 11.16 and 11.17)

- Lymphocytic infiltrate of Jessner

    - Clinical

        ○ Asymptomatic, well-demarcated, erythematous, smooth plaques without surface changes
        ○ Most common on face, but may involve neck and upper extremities

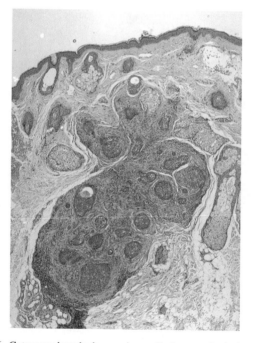

Fig. 11.16 Cutaneous lymphadenoma is a well-circumscribed adnexal tumor with a variable, sometimes dense, lymphocytic infiltrate

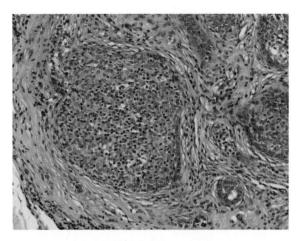

Fig. 11.17 The basaloid lobules of cutaneous lymphadenoma are infiltrated by T and B lymphocytes that lack significant atypia

- o Plaques last for months to years and then usually disappear, but may recur
- o May not represent a discrete entity but may be a *forme fruste* of lupus erythematosus or evolving cutaneous B-cell lymphoma

– Histology

- o Unremarkable epidermis
- o Large aggregates of lymphocytes present in dermis
- o Few plasma cells and histiocytes, but no eosinophils
- o Vague perivascular and peri-appendageal arrangement
- o May extend into subcutaneous fat

– Immunophenotypic analysis

- o No consensus
- o Probably mostly T lymphocytes, with admixture of B cells
- o No lymphocyte surface antigenic abnormalities described (Figs. 11.18, 11.19, 11.20, and 11.21)

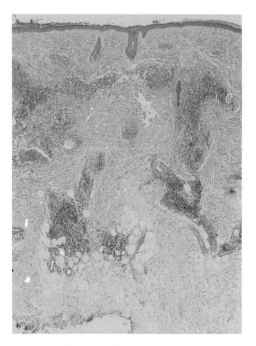

Fig. 11.18 Jessner lymphocytic infiltrate shows a moderately dense perivascular and periadnexal pattern, occasionally with extension into the subcutaneous tissue, as seen here

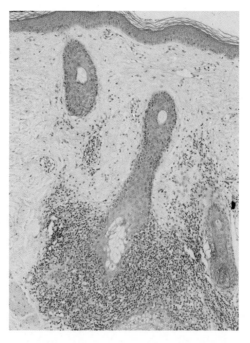

Fig. 11.19 This example of Jessner lymphocytic infiltrate shows predominantly a periadnexal pattern

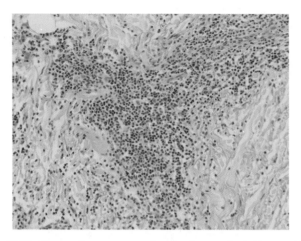

Fig. 11.20 Jessner demonstrates a lymphoplasmacytic infiltrate without neutrophils and eosinophils

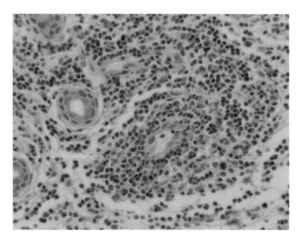

Fig. 11.21 This high-power image of Jessner lymphocytic infiltrate demonstrates the periadnexal pattern and the predominance of lymphocytes and histiocytes with scattered plasma cells

Chapter 12
Dermal Pigmentary Disorders

- Dermal pigmentary disorders

  - Dermal melanin (Table 12.1)

    o Primarily within melanocytes
    o Primarily within melanophages

  - Non-melanin dermal pigment

Table 12.1 Disorders with increased dermal melanin

Blue nevus
Cellular blue nevus
Nevus of Ota
Nevus of Ito
Mongolian spot

- Blue nevus

  - Clinical

    o Blue-black dermal nodule with no overlying epidermal changes
    o Rarely exceeds 1 cm in diameter
    o Often on head and neck or distal extremities
    o Occur in uterine cervix, prostate
    o No predisposition for malignant transformation

B.R. Smoller, K.M. Hiatt, *Inflammatory Dermatoses: The Basics*,
DOI 10.1007/978-1-4419-6004-7_12,
© Springer Science+Business Media, LLC 2010

- Histologic

  - ○ Upper reticular dermis with proliferation of spindle-shaped and dendritic, densely pigmented melanocytes and scattered melanophages
  - ○ May extend into papillary dermis, but no junctional melanocytic proliferation
  - ○ Less pigmented areas and sclerosis in older lesions
  - ○ Unclear etiology –wrests of embryonic melanocytes from below or melanocytes dropping down from the overlying epidermis (Figs. 12.1, 12.2, and 12.3)

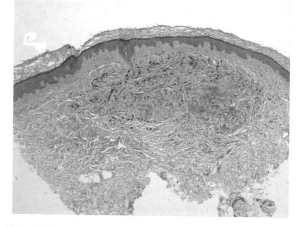

Fig. 12.1 A blue nevus demonstrates abundant melanin in spindle-shaped cells in the upper reticular dermis. Original magnification 40×

- Cellular blue nevus

  - Clinical

    - ○ Majority on buttocks, also common on scalp
    - ○ More common in young to middle-aged women
    - ○ About 1–3 cm diameter
    - ○ Deeply pigmented dermal nodules without overlying surface changes
    - ○ Reports of recurrence and rare malignant degeneration

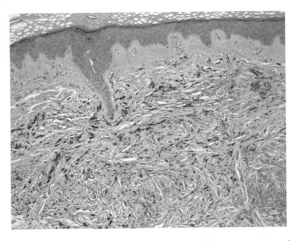

Fig. 12.2 A blue nevus is characterized by spindled melanocytes and more epithelioid-appearing melanophages located in the dermis. Original magnification 100×

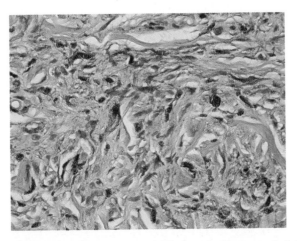

Fig. 12.3 Blue nevi demonstrate a combination of melanocytes (spindled) and melanophages (often epithelioid) that can be best distinguished by cell shape, but cannot always be distinguished. Original magnification 400×

– Histologic

    ○ Biphasic pattern – densely pigmented spindle-shaped cells and nests of plump ovoid cells with virtually no pigment
    ○ Storiform pattern
    ○ May be slight cytologic atypia and rare mitoses
    ○ Junctional melanocytic proliferation would be most unusual
    ○ Zonal necrosis associated with malignant transformation
    ○ *Some histologic overlap with deep penetrating nevus (Volume III)* (Figs. 12.4, 12.5, and 12.6)

• Nevus of Ota

– Clinical

    ○ Unilateral blue-black discoloration of face, especially peri-orbital
    ○ Sclera of eye may also be discolored
    ○ Ten percent bilateral

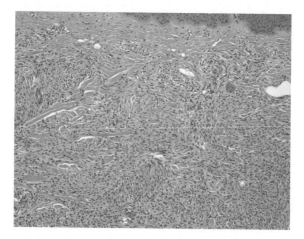

Fig. 12.4 Cellular blue nevi generally spare the epidermis and papillary dermis. A densely cellular spindle-shaped population of melanocytes is present in the reticular dermis. Original magnification 100×

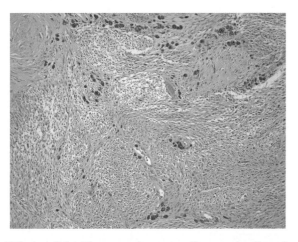

Fig. 12.5 A cellular blue nevus has two cell types: bundles of ovoid melanocytes with little pigment and clusters of densely pigmented melanophages. This cellular lesion often fills the reticular dermis and may extend into the subcutaneous fat. Original magnification 100×

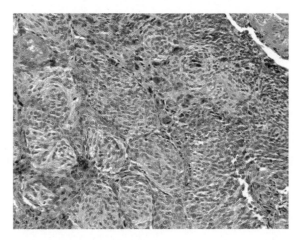

Fig. 12.6 The characteristic biphasic population seen in cellular blue nevi often has an "organoid" appearance. Original magnification 200×

- o Present at birth or early childhood
- o Associated with persistent Mongolian spots

- Histologic

  - o Elongated, spindle-shaped dermal melanocytes in the upper third of the reticular dermis
  - o No junctional melanocytic proliferation
  - o No cytologic atypia, no mitoses
  - o *Histology identical to nevus of Ito*
  - o *More densely populated than Mongolian spot and more superficially located*
  - o Probably a hamartoma of melanocytes (Figs. 12.7 and 12.8)

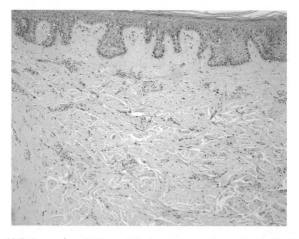

Fig. 12.7 In nevus of Ota, relatively scant numbers of spindle-shaped melanocytes are present within the reticular dermis. Original magnification 100×

- Nevus of Ito

  - Clinical

    - o Located in supraclavicular, scapular, and deltoid regions
    - o Otherwise, identical to nevus of Ota
    - o Mottled, macular appearance

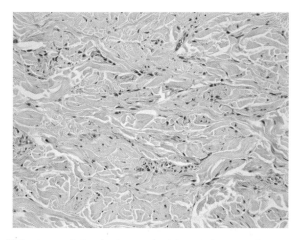

Fig. 12.8 Nevus of Ota is characterized by relatively small numbers of melanocytes coursing between collagen bundles in the reticular dermis. The histologic changes may be quite subtle. Original magnification 200×

- Histologic

  o See nevus of Ota (above) (Fig. 12.9)

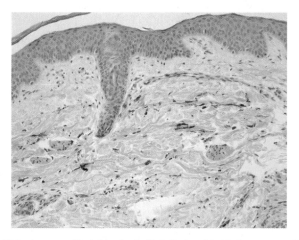

Fig. 12.9 A nevus of Ito is histologically indistinguishable from nevus of Ota. Clinical correlation is essential. Original magnification 200×

- Mongolian spot

  - Clinical

    o Sacrococcygeal
    o Uniform blue discoloration
    o Ill-defined oval patch, resembles a bruise
    o Frequently in non-Caucasian infants; rare in Caucasians
    o Present at birth, disappears within 3–4 years
    o Persists in 3–4% of all patients

  - Histologic

    o Lower reticular dermal infiltrate of elongated, slender dendritic cells with melanin granules
    o No junctional melanocytic proliferation
    o Very paucicellular
    o No melanophages identified
    o Caused by delayed disappearance of dermal melanocytes (not a hamartoma) (Fig. 12.10, Table 12.2)

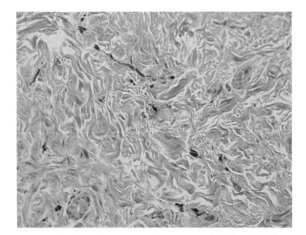

Fig. 12.10 In Mongolian spot, there are even fewer reticular dermal spindle-shaped melanocytes than are in nevus of Ito or Ota. The findings are quite subtle and high magnification is often essential to identify the dermal melanocytes. Original magnification 200×

Table 12.2 Disorders with increased melanophages

Post-inflammatory pigmentary alteration
Chlorpromazine pigmentation
Regression

- Post-inflammatory pigmentary alteration

  - Clinical

    o Consequence of wide range of interface dermatitides characterized by basal vacuolization and keratinocyte disruption
    o Clinically characterized by patterned gray-brown pigmentation that responds very slowly to treatment

  - Histologic

    o Melanophages present in papillary dermis, stain with Fontana stain for melanin, but usually apparent on routine sections
    o May be residual inflammation (lymphocytes)
    o In active lesions, may still see basal vacuolization, dying keratinocytes (Figs. 12.11 and 12.12)

- Post-inflammatory pigmentary alteration

  - Partial differential diagnosis

    o Congenital disorders

      Poikiloderma congenitale
      Xeroderma pigmentosum
      Incontinentia pigmenti

    o Acquired disorders

      Poikiloderma atrophicans vasculare
      Erythema ab igne
      Fixed drug eruption
      Erythema dyschromicum perstans

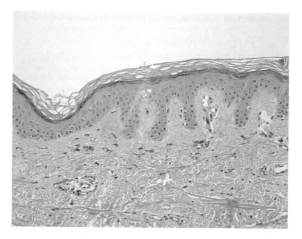

Fig. 12.11 In post-inflammatory pigmentary alteration, clusters of melanophages are present around vessels of the superficial vascular plexus. No residual epidermal changes may be present. Original magnification 200×

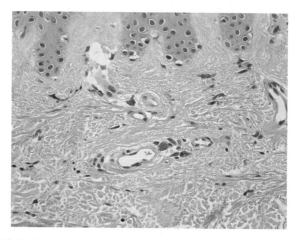

Fig. 12.12 Melanin granules can be identified within the epithelioid pigment-laden macrophages surrounding superficial vessels in post-inflammatory pigmentary alteration. Original magnification 200×

- Chlorpromazine hyperpigmentation

  - Clinical

    o Occurs in 1–15% of patients taking >800 mg/day for >1 year
    o Accentuated with sun exposure
    o More common in women, usually on face
    o Has been reported to involve sclera, cornea, lens

  - Histologic

    o Increased melanin in basal keratinocytes
    o Dark brown granules in macrophages in papillary dermis
    o Negative on Perl's iron stain, positive with Fontana stain for melanin
    o Increased melanosomes in basal keratinocytes form melanin–dechlorinated chlorpromazine polymer complex (Fig. 12.13)

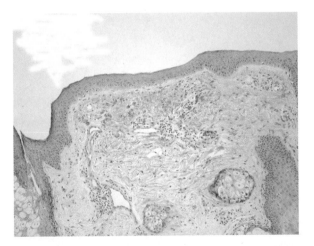

Fig. 12.13 Pigment-laden macrophages are present in the papillary dermis in chlorpromazine hyperpigmentation. Perl's stain for iron (negative) and Fontana stain for melanin (positive) (not shown here) are necessary to confirm the etiology of this pigment. Original magnification 100×

- Regression

  - Clinical

    - Area of hypopigmentation in the region of melanocytic tumor (such as a nevus or a melanoma)
    - May appear scar-like

  - Histologic

    - Atrophic epidermis with flattening of rete ridge pattern
    - Papillary dermal fibrosis (often wispy) with thickening of papillary dermis
    - Increased vascularity
    - Melanophages around superficial vascular plexus
    - Lymphocytic infiltrate
    - May signify previous melanoma or other melanocytic lesion (completely regressed halo nevus) (Figs. 12.14, 12.15, and 12.16, Table 12.3)

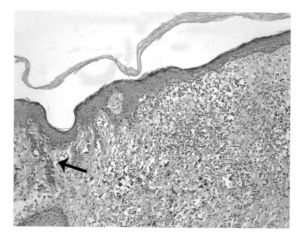

Fig. 12.14 A melanoma (*arrow*) with adjacent regression is seen as characterized by fibrosis, a lymphocytic infiltrate, and scattered dermal melanophages. Original magnification 100×

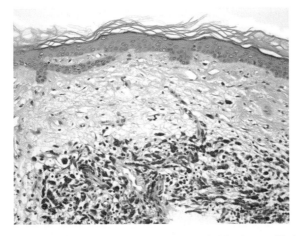

Fig. 12.15 With more extensive regression, there is blunting or ablation of rete ridges by extensive fibrosis and a dense accumulation of melanophages within the dermis. No residual melanocytic proliferation is apparent. Original magnification 200×

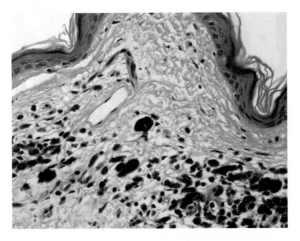

Fig. 12.16 Extensive melanophage accumulation, vascular ectasia, and effacement of rete ridges are present with well-developed, complete regression. Original magnification 400×

Table 12.3 Dermal pigmentary disorders

Dermal pigmentary disorders – non-melanin
Argyria (silver)
Chrysiasis (gold)
Hemosiderosis (iron)
Ochronosis
Amiodarone pigmentation
Tattoo

- Argyria
  - Clinical
    - Must ingest at least 8 g of silver to produce pigmentation
    - Blue to slate-gray discoloration accentuated in sun-exposed areas
    - Gingivae and conjunctivae frequently involved
    - Nails often with similar discoloration

  - Histologic
    - Increased melanin in basal keratinocytes
    - Granules (1 μm) in basal lamina of eccrine ducts, perineurium, and along elastic tissue fibers and collagen bundles
    - Negative with Perl's iron stain and melanin stain
    - Refractile on dark-field examination (Figs. 12.17 and 12.18)

- Chrysiasis
  - Clinical
    - Dose related

      Almost universal with >150 mg/kg
      Most unusual if <50 mg/kg
    - Hyperpigmented only in sun-exposed regions, spares skin folds
    - Pigmentation is irreversible

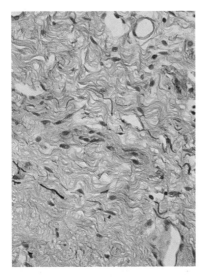

Fig. 12.17 Tiny, pigmented granules are present coating elastic fibers in the dermis in argyria. Original magnification 400×

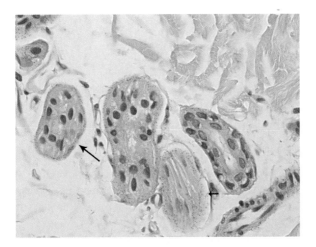

Fig. 12.18 Pigmented granules that are tiny can be found in the lamina propria surrounding eccrine structures in argyria. Original magnification 600×

- Histologic

  - Minimal increase in basal keratinocyte melanin
  - Small, oval black granules present in macrophages, endothelial cells, and basement membranes of eccrine ducts
  - Refractile on dark-field examination
  - *Granules larger than in argyria*

- Hemosideroses

  - Hemochromatosis
  - Minocycline pigmentation
  - Pigmented purpuric eruption (Volume II, Chapter 1)

- Hemochromatosis

  - Clinical

    - Five signs

      Cutaneous hyperpigmentation
      Diabetes mellitus
      Cirrhosis
      Cardiomyopathy
      Arthropathy

    - Gold brown hyperpigmentation accentuated with sun exposure
    - Can be acquired or inherited (autosomal recessive)

  - Histologic

    - Markedly increased melanin in basal keratinocytes
    - Hemosiderin present within macrophages and free in dermis and in basement membrane of eccrine ducts
    - Stains strongly with Perl's iron stain
    - Dermal iron apparently stimulates melanogenesis

- Minocycline hyperpigmentation

  - Clinical

- o Patients on long-term therapy develop blue-black discoloration, especially at sites of scars
- o Partially reversible with cessation of therapy

- Histologic

- o Increased melanin in basal keratinocytes
- o Brown-black granules in macrophages in upper reticular dermis
- o Stains positively with Perl's iron stain and with Fontana–Masson silver stain (like melanin)
- o No melanosomes or premelanosomes in granules on electronic microscopic examination (Figs. 12.19 and 12.20)

- Ochronosis

- Clinical

- o Dark skin, dark urine, arthritis
- o Can be acquired or hereditary (autosomal recessive)

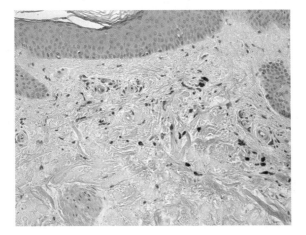

Fig. 12.19 With minocycline-induced hyperpigmentation, pigment-laden macrophages are present surrounding vessels in the superficial vascular plexus. Original magnification 200×

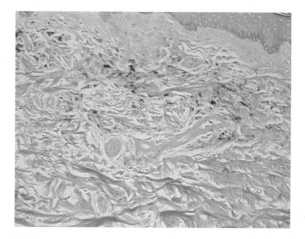

Fig. 12.20 A Perl's stain for iron strongly labels (blue staining) the pigmented cells in minocycline-induced hyperpigmentation. Original magnification 200×

- o Blue-gray pigmentation of cartilage and skin
- o Can have brown sweat
- o Exposure to chemicals such as phenols may induce identical pigmentary changes, but not arthropathy
- o Most commonly encountered in patients using topical bleaching creams for prolonged periods of time

- – Histologic

  - o Yellow-brown granules free in dermis, in macrophages, and in endothelial cells
  - o Large, irregularly shaped granules – can be "ribbon-like"
  - o Deposit around collagen bundles and elastic tissue
  - o Reduce ferric ferricyanide (like melanin), but not silver nitrate (Figs. 12.21 and 12.22)

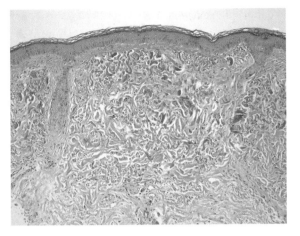

Fig. 12.21 Ochronosis demonstrates large, yellow granules and ribbon-like structures in the superficial dermis. Original magnification 100×

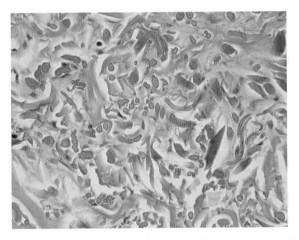

Fig. 12.22 The granules and ribbon-like structures in ochronosis are refractile and *bright yellow*. Original magnification 400×

- Amiodarone pigmentation
  - Clinical
    - Slate blue discoloration with long-term, high-dose therapy in about 10% of cases
    - Pigmentation clinically resembles argyria
  - Histologic
    - Yellow-brown granules in macrophages around vessels of superficial vascular plexus
    - Stains with Fontana–Masson suggesting the presence of melanin and Sudan black suggesting the presence of lipofuscin
    - Perl's iron stain is negative
    - Myelin-like residual bodies seen on electron microscopy within lysosomal granules and in white blood cells

- Tattoo
  - Clinical
    - Black – carbon
    - Blue – cobalt
    - Red – mercuric sulfide
    - Green – chromium
    - Yellow – cadmium sulfide
    - Cadmium added to red to brighten it often results in photoreactions
    - Also can see traumatic graphite tattoos (black)
  - Histologic
    - Pigment located within macrophages surrounding superficial vascular plexus and free in dermis
    - Frequent sarcoidal granulomatous response to pigment (especially red)
    - Professionally done tattoos tend to have pigment located deeper in dermis (Figs. 12.23, 12.24, and 12.25)

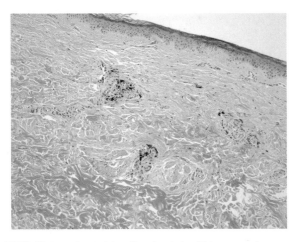

Fig. 12.23 Tattoo pigment is often located within macrophages around dermal blood vessels. Original magnification 100×

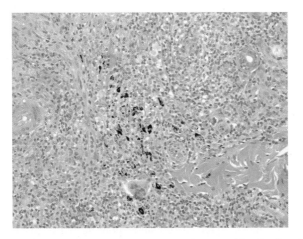

Fig. 12.24 In some tattoos, pigments can be found outside of cells within the dermis, often surrounded by a dense inflammatory and granulomatous response. Original magnification 200×

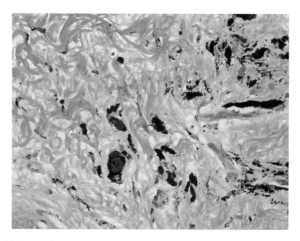

Fig. 12.25 Tattoo pigment may be of many colors, some of which engender a marked host response (not shown here), while others cause virtually none. Original magnification 400×

Chapter 13
Dermal Deposition Disorders Without Pigment

- Amyloidosis

  - Systemic amyloidosis with skin involvement

    o Primary systemic

      Plasma cell dyscrasia produces light chains (AL)
      Deposits may be localized to skin

    o Clinical

      Petechiae and ecchymoses most common on face
      Eyelids frequently involved
      "Pinch purpura" secondary to minor trauma characteristic
        finding
      Macroglossia seen in minority of affected patients

    o Histologic

      Amorphous, eosinophilic masses in dermis and subcutis
      Often in papillary dermis, separated from epidermis by
        only a thin rim of uninvolved dermis
      Fissuring within amyloid deposits is characteristic
      Dense infiltrate of plasma cells often seen surrounding
        amyloid plaques
      Fine needle aspirations of abdominal fat pads will reveal
        amyloid in almost half of all patients with primary
        systemic amyloidosis (Figs. 13.1 and 13.2)

B.R. Smoller, K.M. Hiatt, *Inflammatory Dermatoses: The Basics*,   261
DOI 10.1007/978-1-4419-6004-7_13,
© Springer Science+Business Media, LLC 2010

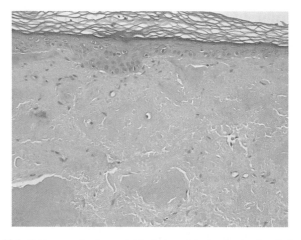

Fig. 13.1 Primary systemic amyloidosis demonstrates sheets of acellular and amorphous eosinophilic material with fissuring within the dermis. Original magnification 200×

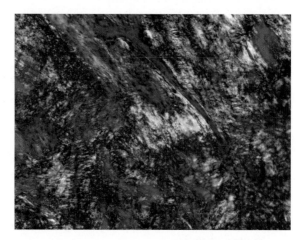

Fig. 13.2 A Congo red stain demonstrates apple green birefringence of the amyloid upon polarization. Original magnification 200×

- Secondary systemic amyloidosis

  o Results from long-standing chronic inflammatory diseases (osteomyelitis, tuberculosis, rheumatoid arthritis)
  o AA amyloid produced
  o No cutaneous lesions as part of this process but amyloid deposits can be found in fat pad aspirates

- Cutaneous amyloidosis

  - Lichen amyloidosis
  - Macular amyloidosis
  - Clinical

    o Probably variations of the same entity
    o *Lichenoid* subtype demonstrates epidermal changes consistent with chronic rubbing including scale, hyperpigmentation, and increased skin markings
    o Red-brown papules with scale that may coalesce into plaques
    o Most common on legs
    o *Macular* subtype with macules in a reticulated pattern
    o Macular subtype is most common on upper back
    o Macular amyloidosis common in Southeast Asia

  - Histologic

    o Lichen amyloidosis

      Hyperkeratosis
      Acanthosis
      Rare dying keratinocytes
      Amorphous to round, eosinophilic deposits in the papillary dermis (size of keratinocytes)
      Relatively scant lymphocytic inflammatory infiltrate
      Eosinophilic deposits in papillary dermis stain with anti-keratin antibodies

    o Macular amyloidosis

      Similar in lichen amyloidosis but without the epidermal changes (Figs. 13.3 and 13.4)

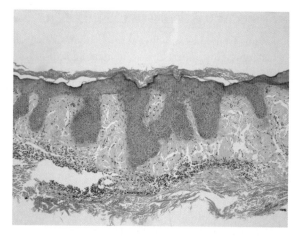

Fig. 13.3 Hyperkeratosis, hypergranulosis, pigmented incontinence, and eosinophilic deposits within the papillary dermis characterize lichen amyloidosis. Original magnification 100×

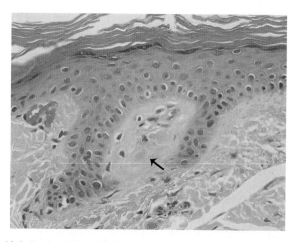

Fig. 13.4 Eosinophilic globules approximately the size of degenerating keratinocytes are present (*arrow*) within the papillary dermis in lichen amyloidosis. Original magnification 400×

- Cutaneous mucinoses

  - Primary
  - Secondary (Table 13.1)

Table 13.1   Primary mucinoses – a histologic classification system

	Increased fibroblasts	Normal numbers of fibroblasts
Superficial mucin	Scleromyxedema Lichen myxedematosus	Pre-tibial myxedema (Generalized myxedema) Focal popular mucinosis
Deep mucin	Nephrogenic systemic fibrosis	Scleredema Pre-tibial myxedema

- Primary mucinoses

  - Scleromyxedema/lichen myxedematosus

    o Clinical

      Waxy 2–3 mm papules on face, extremities
      Lichen myxedematosus – no systemic involvement, skin lesions only
      Scleromyxedema – similar changes but with diffuse thickening of skin and hematologic associations (below)
      Massive involvement of glabellar region may lead to bovine facies
      IgG lambda (usually) paraproteinemia associated with many cases of scleromyxedema
      Similar changes rarely found in viscera and rarely fatal
      Lesions may or may not resolve

    o Histologic

      Epidermis either is unremarkable or demonstrates slight thinning with effacement of rete ridges
      Marked increase in fibroblasts within the superficial reticular dermis

Abundant mucin deposition in superficial reticular dermis that can be highlighted with alcian blue or colloidal iron (pH 4.5)

Slight lymphocytic inflammation (Figs. 13.5, 13.6, and 13.7)

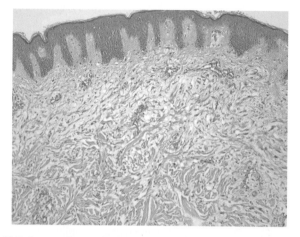

Fig. 13.5 Increased ground substance is present within the upper portion of the reticular dermis along with a noticeable increase in dermal fibroblasts in scleromyxedema. Original magnification 100×

- Nephrogenic systemic fibrosis

  - Clinical

    - Symmetrical thickening of skin primarily on extremities, most commonly lower extremities, that clinically resembles scleroderma
    - Surface of skin is shiny, smooth, and atrophic appearing
    - Usually spares face
    - Always associated with some degree of renal dysfunction
    - Contrast media, such as gadolinium, currently implicated in pathogenesis

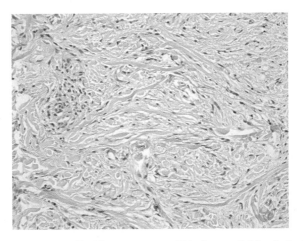

Fig. 13.6 Abundant fibroblasts are present within the superficial reticular dermis in scleromyxedema. A *slight bluish tinge* is present within the background stroma, suggesting increased mucin deposits. Original magnification 200×

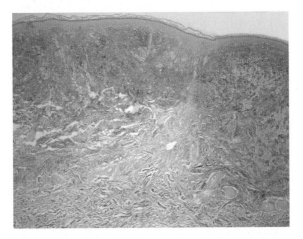

Fig. 13.7 Colloidal iron stain (pH 4.5) demonstrates abundant mucin deposits in the superficial dermis in scleromyxedema. Original magnification 40×

- Histologic

  - ○ Increased numbers of fibroblasts and collagen throughout reticular dermis, with a prevalence for the deep dermis
  - ○ In some cases, extends into subcutaneous fat along the septae
  - ○ Increased amounts of mucin within reticular dermis, extending down into fibrous septa of subcutis in some cases
  - ○ May involve superficial reticular dermis and/or papillary dermis, but this is less common
  - ○ Variably intense lymphocytic inflammatory response
  - ○ *Similar appearance to scleromyxedema except for the involvement of the deeper dermis and subcutis (not seen in scleromyxedema)* (Figs. 13.8 and 13.9)

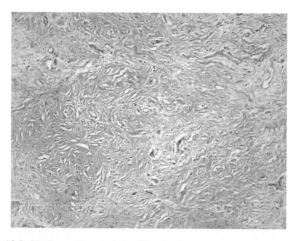

Fig. 13.8 Nephrogenic systemic fibrosis demonstrates increased dermal mucin and fibroblasts in the deeper reticular dermis. Original magnification 100×

- Pre-tibial myxedema

  - Clinical

    - ○ Waxy plaques and nodules with yellowish coloring

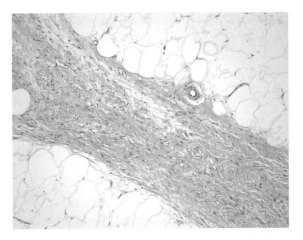

Fig. 13.9 The changes extend into the fibrous septa within the subcutaneous fat in nephrogenic systemic fibrosis. Original magnification 100×

- o Most common on shins and dorsa of feet
- o May involve forearms less commonly
- o Occurs in setting of hyperthyroidism and in association with exophthalmos

- – Histologic

  - o Unremarkable epidermis, occasionally slightly acanthotic
  - o Mucin accumulates in the upper half of the reticular dermis
  - o Mild infiltrate of lymphocytes and mast cells
  - o *Minimal increase in numbers of dermal fibroblasts (as opposed to scleromyxedema)* (Figs. 13.10 and 13.11)

- • Scleredema

  - – Clinical

    - o Two subtypes

      Associated with *Streptococcus pneumoniae* – reversible and more common in children

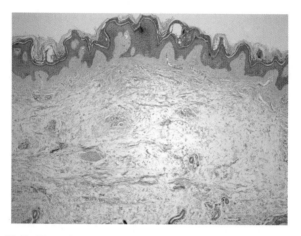

Fig. 13.10 There is an area of pallor in the superficial portion of the reticular dermis, suggesting increased mucin in pre-tibial myxedema. Original magnification 40×

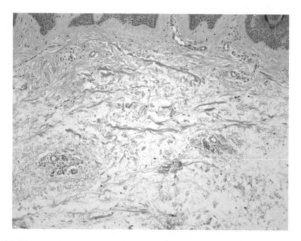

Fig. 13.11 Pre-tibial myxedema is characterized by increased dermal mucin in the upper half of the reticular dermis without an appreciable increase in the numbers of dermal fibroblasts. Original magnification 100×

Associated with diabetes mellitus – irreversible and
almost exclusively in middle-aged to elderly adults
Markedly thickened dermis on back, shoulders, neck
Indurated or waxy plaques
Clinically may resemble scleroderma

- Histologic

  o Normal epidermis
  o Marked thickening of dermis
  o Slightly thickened collagen bundles
  o Increased space (usually clear on routine sections)
    between collagen bundles in reticular dermis
  o Colloidal iron (pH 4.5) demonstrates increased mucin in
    reticular dermis
  o No increase in dermal fibroblasts
  o No associated inflammatory response
  o *Subtle findings – difficult to distinguish from normal
    skin. Clues include marked thickening of total reticular
    dermis and increased spaces between collagen bundles*
    (Figs. 13.12, 13.13, and 13.14)

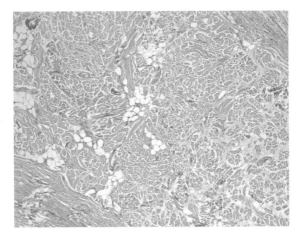

Fig. 13.12 The findings in scleredema are quite subtle. The dermis is
thickened within slight thickening of reticular dermal collagen bundles and
increased interstitial spaces that contain mucin (that is rarely apparent with
routine stains). Original magnification 40×

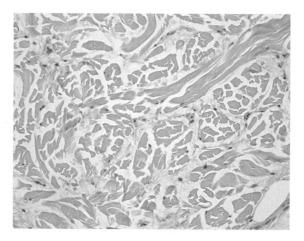

Fig. 13.13 Increased interstitial spaces make collagen bundles appear widely separated in scleredema. There is no increase in dermal cellularity. Original magnification 400×

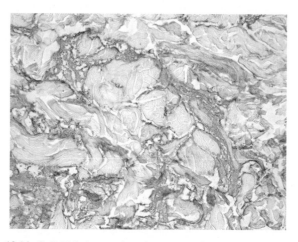

Fig. 13.14 Colloidal iron stains demonstrate increased dermal mucin throughout the entire reticular dermis in scleredema. Original magnification 200×

- Secondary mucinoses

  - Digital mucous cyst
  - Ganglion cyst
  - (Follicular mucinosis – see Volume IV – cutaneous T-cell lymphoma)

- Digital mucous cyst

  - Clinical

    o – Misnomer – not really a "cyst" – accumulation of mucin without a cyst lining
    o Caused by either overproduction of mucin by dermal fibroblasts or underdegradation of the ground substance
    o Dermal nodule located near the proximal nail fold

  - Histologic

    o Poorly circumscribed collection of mucin (acid mucopolysaccharides) in dermis
    o Some cases with increased number of dermal fibroblasts
    o Inflammatory response variable
    o No cyst lining present (Figs. 13.15, 13.16, and 13.17)

- Ganglion cyst

  - Clinical

    o Most common overlying the synovial space in wrist
    o Probably post-traumatic in most cases
    o Cystic nodule without surface changes

  - Histologic

    o Collection of mucin (acid mucopolysaccharides) in deep dermis
    o Often difficult to find residual synovial cyst lining
    o Variable inflammation

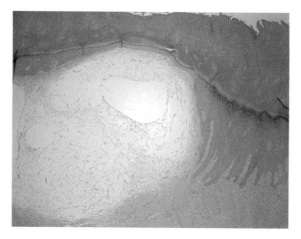

Fig. 13.15 A digital mucous cyst contains a sharply circumscribed but not encapsulated accumulation of dermal mucin on acral skin. Original magnification 40×

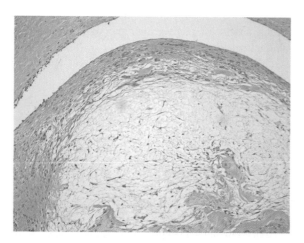

Fig. 13.16 There is no cyst lining in digital mucous cysts, simply a collection of fibroblasts and abundant mucin. Original magnification 100×

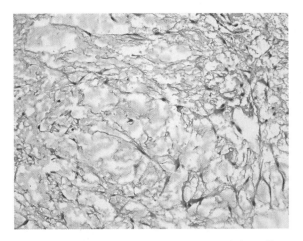

Fig. 13.17 In most digital mucous cysts, the dermal mucin is readily apparent on routine stains and stains for acid mucopolysaccharides are not necessary. Original magnification 200×

- Colloid milium/nodular elastosis (Table 13.2)

Table 13.2 Types of colloid milium

Adult type
Nodular colloid degeneration
Juvenile type

- Clinical
  - Adult type

    Involves face, neck, and dorsal hands
    Related to sun exposure

  - Nodular colloid degeneration

    One or several nodules on face, scalp
    Apparently unrelated to sun exposure

   o Juvenile type

     Onset prior to puberty
     Waxy, brown papules mainly on face
     Related to sun exposure
     Most cases with family history of colloid milium

– Histologic

   o Adult type

     Epidermis normal or slightly thinned
     Papillary dermis uninvolved
     Reticular dermis filled with amorphous masses of fissured pink-gray material
     Minimal cellularity in dermis

   o Nodular colloid degeneration

     Flattened epidermis
     Papillary and reticular dermis filled with gray-pink amorphous material
     Minimal accompanying infiltrate of fibroblasts

   o Juvenile type

     Colloid is derived from keratinocytes
     Flattened rete ridges
     Basal cells with focal degeneration
     "Parched pavement" appearance – gray masses of material with fissures
     Amorphous masses stain with anti-keratin antibodies, unlike nodular colloid degeneration or adult-type colloid milium
     All three types of colloid milium difficult to distinguish from amyloidosis: Congo red positive (weakly), fluorescent with thioflavin T, and PASD positive (Figs. 13.18 and 13.19)

• Collagen

– Nephrogenic systemic fibrosis (see above)
– Scleroderma

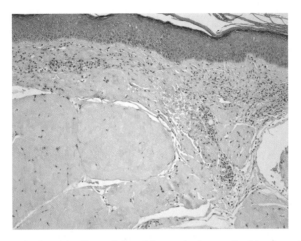

Fig. 13.18 Colloid milium of the adult type is characterized by amorphous *pink-gray* masses of acellular material separated from the epidermis by a small zone of sparing. Original magnification 100×

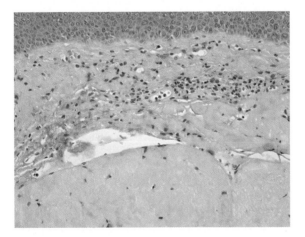

Fig. 13.19 The masses of amorphous material in colloid milium may be fissured and may strongly resemble amyloidosis in the skin. Original magnification 200×

o Clinical

   Localized and systemic variants

   Localized is seen primarily in children and young adults, females more commonly than males

   Indurated plaque with a shiny center and a violaceous border

   Systemic variant is progressive and presents with symmetric thickening of the skin

   Associated with CREST syndrome when there is limited disease

o Histologic

   Epidermis may be atrophic, hypertrophic, or normal

   Dermis is thickened with increased collagen that is characterized by thickened bundles

   No significant increase in fibroblasts

   Collagen deposition replaces peri-adnexal fat

   Follicles may be obliterated and arrector pili muscles are typically hypertrophic

   May displace eccrine glands into the mid-dermis

   A mild lymphoplasmacytic inflammatory infiltrate may be present around the vessels and at the base of the collagen deposition

   The dense collagen results in a characteristic straight, abrupt edge at the biopsy margin (Fig. 13.20)

- Calcification and ossification

  – Calcinosis cutis (Table 13.3)

Table 13.3 Calcinosis cutis

Calcinosis universalis associated with dermatomyositis
Tumoral calcinosis
Subepidermal calcified nodule
Idiopathic scrotal calcinosis
Dystrophic calcification
Metastatic calcification

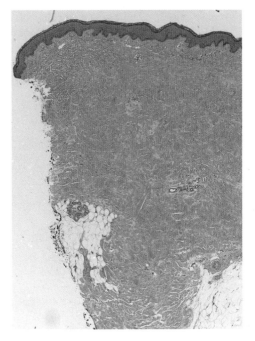

Fig. 13.20 This example of morphea shows dense dermal collagen with atrophy of the adnexal structures. Note the location of the eccrine gland in the dermis and the unusually straight borders to the biopsy

- Clinical

  - o Dermal nodules with minimal surface change
  - o Rarely ulcerate
  - o Can be in many locations
  - o Metastatic calcification associated with hyperparathyroidism and hypervitaminosis D

- Histologic

  - o Foci of calcium within dermis
  - o May be surrounded by inflammatory infiltrate and occasionally granulomas

- o Dystrophic etiologies often have residue of antecedent folliculitis or other locally destructive inflammatory processes
- o von Kossa stain can be used to highlight calcium (rarely needed) or alizarin red to identify phosphate in calcium phosphate deposits (Figs. 13.21 and 13.22)

- Osteoma cutis

  – Clinical

    - o Dermal and/or subcutaneous nodules
    - o Often associated with long-standing acne vulgaris or other chronic inflammatory processes
    - o Faces of young women frequently affected (secondary to acne vulgaris)

  – Histologic

    - o Small foci of well-formed bone are present within the dermis

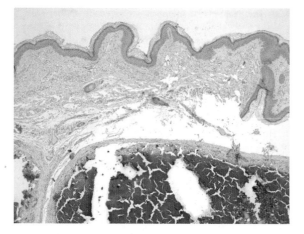

Fig. 13.21 *Purple* masses with marked fracturing within the dermis characterize the changes in calcinosis cutis (in this case, idiopathic scrotal calcinosis). Original magnification 40×

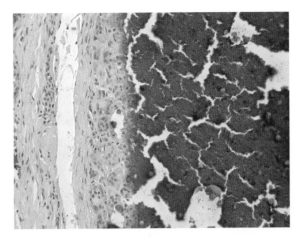

Fig. 13.22 A granulomatous and giant cell reaction is often present surrounding calcium deposits in calcinosis cutis. Original magnification 200×

- o Often located near hair follicles
- o Marrow spaces may be present and include extramedullary hematopoiesis (Figs. 13.23 and 13.24)

- Lipoid proteinosis (hyalinosis cutis et mucosae)

  - Clinical

    - o Very rare
    - o Papules and nodules on face with overlying hyperpigmentation
    - o Involvement of extremities less common
    - o Papules along edges of eyelids – very characteristic
    - o Thickened tongue
    - o Involvement of vocal cords leads to hoarseness
    - o Caused by mutation in extracellular matrix protein 1 (*ECM1*) gene

  - Histologic

    - o Acellular, eosinophilic material present around capillaries and within lamina propria of eccrine apparatus

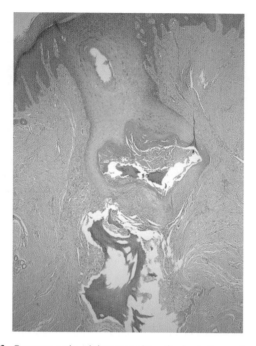

Fig. 13.23 Osteoma cutis originates at sites of prior inflammation in many cases (in this section it is seen at the site of a previous folliculitis). Original magnification 40×

- o Similar "hyaline-like" material in papillary dermis
- o Material is PASD positive and may stain slightly with colloidal iron at pH 2.5 (Figs. 13.25 and 13.26)

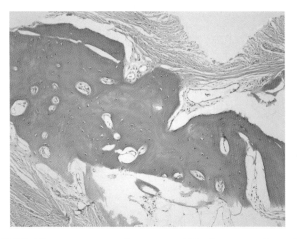

Fig. 13.24 Marrow spaces may be present within the masses of osteoid in osteoma cutis. Original magnification 100×

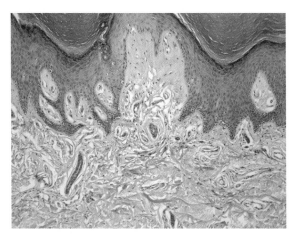

Fig. 13.25 Amorphous and acellular masses of eosinophilic material are present within the papillary dermis in lipoid proteinosis (hyalinosis cutis et mucosae). Original magnification 100×

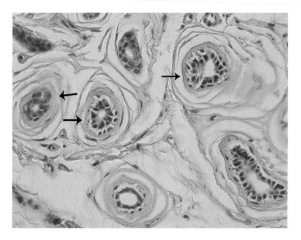

Fig. 13.26 Eosinophilic material deposits within the lamina propria of eccrine structures (*arrows*) in lipoid proteinosis. Original magnification 400×

Further Reading

Chapter 1

Pigmented Purpuric Eruption

Magro CM, Schaefer JT, Crowson AN, Li J, Morrison C. Pigmented purpuric dermatoses. Am J Clin Pathol 2007; 128: 218–229.

Puddin P, Ferranti G, Frezzolini A, Colonna L, Cianchini G. Pigmented purpura-like eruption as a cutaneous sign f mycosis fungoides with autoimmune purpura. J Am Acad Dermatol 1999; 40: 298–299.

Randall SJ, Kierland RR, Montgomery H. Pigmented purpuric eruptions. AMA Arch Derm Syphilol 1951; 64: 177–191.

Viral Exanthem

Drago F, Rampini E, Rebora A. Atypical exanthems: morphology and laboratory investigations may lead to an aetiological diagnosis in about 70% of cases. Br J Dermatol 2002; 147: 255–260.

Mays SR, Kunishige JH, Truong E, Kontoyiannis DP, Hymes SR. Approach to the morbilliform eruption in the hematopoietic

B.R. Smoller, K.M. Hiatt, *Inflammatory Dermatoses: The Basics*, 285
DOI 10.1007/978-1-4419-6004-7,
© Springer Science+Business Media, LLC 2010

transplant patient. Semin Cutan Med Surg 2007; 26: 155–162.

Gyrate Erythema

Weyers W, Diaz-Cascajo C, Weyers I. Erythema annulare centrifugum: results of a clinicopathologic study of 73 patients. Am J Dermatopathol 2003; 25: 451–462.

Ziemer M, Eisendle K, Zelger B. New concepts on erythema annulare centrifugum: a clinical reaction pattern that does not represent a specific Clinicopathologic entity. Br J Dermatol 2009; 160: 119–126.

Post-inflammatory Pigmentary Alteration

Rocky Mountain Spotted Fever

Chen LF, Sexton DJ. What's new in Rocky Mountain spotted fever? Infect Dis Clin North Am 2008; 45: 741–744.

Kao GF, Evancho CD, Joffe O, Lowitt MH, Dumler JS. Cutaneous histopathology of Rocky Mountain spotted fever. J Cutan Pathol 1997; 24: 604–610.

Kim J, Smith KJ, Naefie R, Skelton H. Histopathologic features of and lymphoid populations in the skin of patients with the spotted fever group of rickettsiae: southern Africa. Int J Dermatol 2004; 43: 188–194.

Polymorphous Light Eruption

Dummer R, Ivanova K, Scheidegger EP, Burg G. Clinical and therapeutic aspects of polymorphous light eruption. Dermatology 2003; 207: 93–95.

Epstein JH. Polymorphous light eruption. J Am Acad Dermatol 1980; 3: 329–343.

Naleway AL. Polymorphous light eruption. Int J Dermatol 2002; 41: 377–383.

Urticaria

Fung MA. The clinical and histopathologic spectrum of "dermal hypersensitivity reactions," a non-specific histologic diagnosis that is not very useful in clinical practice, and the concept of a "dermal hypersensitivity reaction pattern". J Am Acad Dermatol 2002; 47: 898–907.

Jordaan HF, Schneider JW. Papular urticaria: a histologic study of 30 patients. Am J Dermatopathol 1997; 19: 119–126.

Kossard S, Hammann I, Wilkinson B. Defining urticarial dermatitis. Arch Dermatol 2996; 142: 29–34.

Arthropod Bite Reactions

Millikan LE. Papular urticaria. Semin Dermatol 1993; 12: 53–56.

Steen CJ, Carbonaro PA, Schwarz RA. Arthropods in dermatology. J Am Acad Dermatol 2004; 40: 819–842.

Pruritic Urticarial Papules and Plaques of Pregnancy

Aronson IK, Bond S, Fiedler VC, Vomvouras S, Gruber D, Ruiz C. Pruritic urticarial papules and plaques of pregnancy: clinical and immunopathologic observations in 57 patients. J Am Acad Dermatol 1998; 39: 933–939.

Callen JP, Hann R. Pruritic urticarial papules and plaques of pregnancy (PUPPP). A clinicopathologic study. J Am Acad Dermatol 1981; 5: 401–405.

Cohen LM, Capeless EL. Krusinski PA, Maloney ME. Pruritic urticarial papules and plaques of pregnancy and its relationship to maternal-fetal weight gain and twin pregnancy. Arch Dermatol 1989; 125: 1534–1536.

Matz H, Orion E, Wolf R. Pruritic urticarial papules and plaques of pregnancy: polymorphic eruption of pregnancy (PUPPP). Clin Dermatol 2006; 24: 105–108.

Chapter 2

Erythema Multiforme

Bastuji-Garin S, Rzany B, Stern RS, Shear NH, Naldi L, Roujeau J-C. Clinical classification of cases of toxic epidermal necrolysis, Stevens–Johnson syndrome and erythema multiforme. Arch Dermatol 1993; 129: 92–96.

Huff JC, Weston WL, Tonnesen MG. Erythema multiforme: a critical review of characteristics, diagnostic criteria and causes. J Am Acad Dermatol 1983; 8: 763–775.

Reed RJ. Erythema multiforme. A clinical syndrome and a histologic complex. Am J Dermatopathol 1985; 7: 143–152.

Zohdi-Mofid M, Horn TD. Acrosyringeal concentration of necrotic keratinocytes in erythema multiforme: a clue to drug etiology. Clinicopathologic review of 29 cases. J Cutan Pathol 1997; 24: 235–240.

Graft Vs. Host Disease

Ferrara JLM, Deeg HJ. Graft-vs-host disease. N Engl J Med 1991; 324: 667–674.

Hood AF, Vogelsang GB, Black LP, Farmer ER, Santos GW. Acute graft-vs-host disease: development following autologous and syngeneic bone marrow transplantation. Arch Dermatol 1987; 123: 745–750.

Zhou Y, Barnett MJ, Rivers JK. Clinical significance of skin biopsies in the diagnosis and management of graft-vs-host disease in early post-allogeneic bone marrow transplantation. Arch Dermatol 2000; 136: 717–721.

Lupus Erythematosus

Bangert J, Freeman R, Sontheimer RD, Gilliam JN. Subacute cutaneous lupus erythematosus and discoid lupus erythematosus. Comparative histologic findings. Arch Dermatol 1984; 120: 332–337.

Bielsam I, Gerrero C, Collado A, Cobos A, Palou J, Mascaro JM. Histopathologic findings in cutaneous lupus erythematosus. Arch Dermatol 1994; 130: 54–58.

Harrist TJ, Mihm MC, Jr. The specificity and clinical usefulness of the lupus band test. Arthritis Rheum 1980; 23: 479–490.

Jerden MS, Hood AF, Moore GW, Callen JP. Histopathologic comparison of the subsets of lupus erythematosus. Arch Dermatol 1990; 126: 52–55.

Dermatomyositis

Callen JP. Dermatomyositis. Dermatol Clin 1983; 1: 461–473.

Jorizzo LR 3rd, Jorizzo JL. The treatment and prognosis of dermatomyositis: an updated review. J Am Acad Dermatol 2008; 59: 99–112.

Tymms DE, Webb J. Dermatomyositis and other connective tissue disease: a review of 105 cases. J Rheumatol 1985; 12: 1140–1148.

Lichen Sclerosus

Carlson JA, Lamb P, Malfetano J, Ambros RA, Mihm MC, Jr. Clinicopathologic comparison of vulvar and extragenital lichen sclerosus: histologic variants, evolving lesions, and etiology of 141 cases. Mod Pathol 1998; 11: 844–854.

Fung MA, LeBoit PE. Light microscopic criteria for the diagnosis of early vulvar lichen sclerosus: a comparison with lichen planus. Am J Surg Pathol 1998; 22: 473–478.

Radiation Dermatitis

Hymes SR, Strom EA, Fife C. Radiation dermatitis: clinical pre-
    sentation, pathophysiology, and treatment 2006. J Am Acad
    Dermatol 2006; 54: 28–46.

Pityriasis Lichenoides Chronica

Magro C, Crowson AN, Kovatich A, Burns E. Pityriasis
    lichenoides: a clonal T-cell lymphoproliferative disorder. Hum
    Pathol 2002; 33: 788–795.
Rogers M. Pityriasis lichenoides and lymphomatoid papulosis.
    Semin Dermatol 1992; 11: 73–79.
Romani J, Puig L, Fernandez-Figueras MT, de Moragas JM.
    Pityriasis lichenoides in children: clinicopathologic review of
    22 patients. Pediatr Dermatol 1998; 15: 1–6.

Lichen Planus

Boyd AS. Update on the diagnosis of lichenoid dermatitis. Adv
    Dermatol 1996; 11: 287–315.
Oliver GF, Winkelmann RK, Muller SA. Lichenoid dermatitis: a
    clinicopathologic and immunopathologic review of sixty-two
    cases. J Am Acad Dermatol 1989; 21: 284–292.
Patel GK, Turner RJ, Marks R. Cutaneous lichen planus and squa-
    mous cell carcinoma. J Eur Acad Dermatol Venereol 2003; 17:
    98–100.

Lichenoid Drug Eruption

Halvey S, Shai A. Lichenoid drug eruption. J Am Acad Dermatol
    1993; 29: 249–255.
Shiohara T, Mizukawa Y. The immunologic basis of lichenoid
    tissue reaction. Autoimmun Rev 2005; 4: 236–241.

Van de Haute V, Antoine JL, Lachapelle JM. Histopathological discriminant criteria between lichenoid drug eruption and idiopathic lichen planus: retrospective study on selected samples. Dermatologica 1989; 179: 10–13.

Lichenoid Keratosis

Miteva M, Ziemer M. Lichenoid keratosis: a clinicopathologic entity with lupus erythematosus-like features? J Cutan Pathol 2007; 34: 209–210.

Morgan MB, Stevens GL, Switlyk S. Benign lichenoid keratosis: a clinical and pathologic reappraisal of 1040 cases. Am J Dermatopathol 2005; 27: 387–392.

Prieto VG, Casal M, McNutt NS. Immunohistochemistry detects differences between lichen planus-like keratosis, lichen planus and lichenoid actinic keratosis. J Cutan Pathol 1993; 20: 143–147.

Lichen Striatus

Patrizi A, Neri I, Fiorentini C, Bonci A, Ricci G. Lichen striatus: clinical and laboratory features of 115 children. Pediatr Dermatol 2004; 21: 197–204.

Permiquel L, Baselga E, Dalmau J, Roe E, del Mar Campos M, Alomar A. Lichen striatus: clinical and epidemiologic review of 23 cases. Eur J Pediatr 2006; 165: 267–269.

Zhang Y, McNutt NS. Lichen striatus: histological, immunohistochemical and ultrastructural study of 57 cases. J Cutan Pathol 2001; 28: 65–71.

Lichen Nitidus

Tilly JJ, Drolet BA, Easterly NB. Lichenoid eruptions in children. J Am Acad Dermatol 2004; 51: 606–624.

Chapter 3

Contact Dermatitis

Cohen DE. Contact dermatitis: a quarter century perspective. J Am Acad Dermatol 2005: 1(1 Suppl); S60–S63.

Wildemore JK, Junkins-Hopkins JM, James WD. Evaluation of the histologic characteristics of patch test confirmed allergic contact dermatitis. J Am Acad Dermatol 2003; 49: 243–248.

Dermatophyte

Loos DS. Cutaneous fungal infections in the elderly. Dermatol Clin 2004; 22: 33–50.

Weitzman I, Padhye AA. Dermatophytes: gross and microscopic. Dermatol Clin 1996; 14: 9–22.

Pityriasis Rosea

Chuh AA, Chan HH, Zawar V. Is human herpesvirus 7 the causative agent of pityriasis rosea? A critical review. Int J Dermatol 2004; 43: 870–875.

Gonzalez LM, Allen R, Janniger CK, Schwartz RA. Pityriasis rosea: an important papulosquamous disorder. Int J Dermatol 2005; 44: 757–764.

Parson JM. Pityriasis rosea: update: 1986. J Am Acad Dermatol 1986; 15: 159–167.

Photo-allergic Drug Eruptions

Gonzalez E, Gonzalez S. Drug photosensitivity, idiopathic photodermatoses and sunscreens. J Am Acad Dermatol 1996; 35: 871–885.

Yashar SS, Lim HW. Classification and evaluation of photodermatoses. Dermatol Ther 2003; 16: 1–7.

Chapter 4

Psoriasis

Murphy M, Kerr P, Grant-Kels JM. The histopathologic spectrum of psoriasis. Clin Dermatol 2007; 25: 524–528.

Naldi L, Gambini D. The clinical spectrum of psoriasis. Clin Dermatol 2007; 25: 510–518.

Nickoloff BJ, Qin JZ, Nestle FO. Immunopathogenesis of psoriasis. Clin Rev Allergy Immunol 2007: 33: 45–56.

Seborrheic Dermatitis

Fox BJ, Odam RB. Papulosquamous diseases: a review. J Am Acad Dermatol 1985; 12: 597–624.

Houck G, Saeed S, Stevens GL, Morgan MB. Eczema and the spongiotic dermatoses: a histologic and pathogenic update. Semin Cutan Med Surg 2004; 23: 39–45.

Secondary Syphilis

Jordaan HF. Secondary syphilis. A clinicopathologic study. Am J Dermatopathol 1988; 10: 399–409.

Jordaan HF, Louw M. The moth-eaten alopecia of secondary syphilis. A histopathologic study of 12 patients. Am J Dermatopathol 1995; 17: 158–162.

Lichen Simplex Chronicus

Gunasti S, Marakli SS, Tuncer I, Ozpoyraz N, Aksungur VL. Clinical and histopathological findings of 'psoriatic neurodermatitis' and of typical lichen simplex chronicus. J Eur Acad Dermatol Venereol 2007; 21: 811–817.

Pityriasis Rubra Pilaris

Albert MR, Mackool BT. Pityriasis rubra pilaris. Int J Dermatol 1999; 38: 1–11.

Magro CM, Crowson AN. The clinical and histomorphological features of pityriasis rubra pilaris. A comparative analysis with psoriasis. J Cutan Pathol 1997; 24: 416–424.

Chapter 5

Epidermolysis Bullosa

Fine JD, Eady RA, Bauer EA, Bauer JW, Bruckner-Tuderman L, Heagety A, Hintner H, Hovnanian A, Jonkman MF, Leigh I, McGrath JA, Mellerio JE, Murrell DF, Shimizu H, Uitto J, Valquist A, Woodley D, Zambrano G. The classification of inherited epidermolysis bullosa (EB): report of the Third International Consensus Meeting on Diagnosis and Classification of EB. J Am Acad Dermatol 2008; 58: 931–950.

McAllister JC, Marinkovich P. Advances in inherited epidermolysis bullosa. Adv Dermatol 2005; 21: 303–334.

Porphyria Cutanea Tarda

Meola T, Lim HW. The porphyrias. Dermatol Clin 1993; 11: 583–596.

Touart DM, Sau P. Cutaneous deposition diseases. Part I. J Am Acad Dermatol 1998; 39: 149–171.

Polymorphous Light Eruption

Honigsman H. Polymorphous light eruption. Photodermatol Photoimmunol Photomed 2008; 24: 155–161.

Naleway AL. Polymorphous light eruption. Int J Dermatol 2002; 41: 377–383.

Bullous Pemphigoid

Kasperkiewicz M, Zillikens D. The pathophysiology of bullous pemphigoid. Clin Rev Allergy Immunology 2007; 33: 78–84.

Kolanko E, Bickle K, Keehn C, Glass LE. Subepidermal blistering disorders: a clinical and histopathologic review. Semin Cutan Med Surg 2004; 23: 10–18.

Liu Z, Diaz LA. Bullous pemphigoid: end of the century review. J Dermatol 2001; 28: 647–650.

Pemphigoides (Herpes) Gestationis

Engineer L, Bhol K, Ahmed AR. Pemphigoid gestationis: a review. Am J Obstet Gynecol 2000; 183: 483–491.

Kolanko E, Bickle K, Keehn C, Glass LE. Subepidermal blistering disorders: a clinical and histopathologic review. Semin Cutan Med Surg 2004; 23: 10–18.

Shornick JK. Herpes gestationis. Dermatol Clin 1993; 11: 527–533.

Dermatitis Herpetiformis

Alonso-Llamazares J, Gibson LE, Rogers RS 3rd. Clinical, pathologic, and immunopathologic features of dermatitis herpetiformis: review of the Mayo Clinic experience. Int J Dermatol 2007; 46: 910–919.

Fry L. Dermatitis herpetiformis: problems, progress and prospects. Eur J Dermatol 2002; 12: 523–531.

Nicolas ME, Krause PK, Gibson LE, Murray JA. Dermatitis herpetiformis. Int J Dermatol 2003: 42: 588–600.

Linear IgA Bullous Dermatitis (Bullous Dermatosis of Childhood)

Egan CA, Zone JJ. Linear IgA bullous dermatosis. Int J Dermatol 1999; 38: 818–827.
Guide SV, Marinkovich MP. Linear IgA bullous dermatosis. Clin Dermatol 2001; 19: 719–727.
Onodera H, Mihm MC, Jr., Yoshida A, Akasaka T. Drug-induced linear IgA bullous dermatosis. J Dermatol 2005; 32: 759–764.

Bullous Urticaria Pigmentosa

Hartmann K, Metcalfe DD. Pediatric mastocytosis. Hematol Oncol Clin North Am 2000; 14: 625–640.
Soter NA. Mastocytosis and the skin. Hematol Oncol Clin North Am 2000; 14: 537–555.
Wolff K, Komar M, Petzelbauer P. Clinical and histopathological aspects of cutaneous mastocytosis. Leuk Res 2001; 25: 519–528.

Chapter 6

Epidermolysis Bullosa Simplex

Fine JD, Eady RA, Bauer EA, Bauer JW, Bruckner-Tuderman L, Heagety A, Hintner H, Hovnanian A, Jonkman MF, Leigh I, McGrath JA, Mellerio JE, Murrell DF, Shimizu H, Uitto J, Valquist A, Woodley D, Zambrano G. The classification of inherited epidermolysis bullosa (EB): report of the Third International Consensus Meeting on Diagnosis and Classification of EB. J Am Acad Dermatol 2008; 58: 931–950.
McAllister JC, Marinkovich P. Advances in inherited epidermolysis bullosa. Adv Dermatol 2005; 21: 303–334.

Pemphigus Vulgaris

Baroni A, Lanza A, Cirillo N, Brunetti G, Ruocco E, Ruocco V. Vesicular and bullous disorders: pemphigus. Dermatol Clin 2007; 25: 597–603.

Hashimoto T. Recent advances in the study of the pathophysiology of pemphigus. Arch Dermatol Res 2003; 295(Suppl 1): S2–S11.

Pemphigus Vegetans

Becker BA, Gaspari AA. Pemphigus vulgaris and vegetans. Dermatol Clin 1993; 11: 429–452.

Paraneoplastic Pemphigus

Anhalt GJ. Paraneoplastic pemphigus. J Invest Dermatol Symp Proc 2004; 9: 29–33.

Anhalt GJ. Paraneoplastic pemphigus. Adv Dermatol 1997; 12: 77–96.

Hailey-Hailey Disease

Chidgey M. Desmosomes and disease: an update. Histol Histopathol 2002; 17: 1179–1192.

McGrath JA. Hereditary diseases of desmosomes. J Dermatol Sci 1999; 20: 85–91.

Darier's Disease

Burge S. Darier's disease – the clinical features and pathogenesis. Clin Exp Dermatol 1994; 19: 193–205.

Sehgal VN, Srivastava G. Darier's (Darier–White) disease/keratosis follicularis. Int J Dermatol 2005; 44: 184–192.

Grover's Disease (*Transient* Acantholytic *Dermatosis*)

Davis MD, Dineen AM, Landa N, Gibson LE. Grover's disease: clinicopathologic review of 72 cases. Mayo Clin Proc 1999; 74: 229–234.

Hashimoto K, Fujiwara K, Tada J, Harada M, Setoyama M, Eto H. Desmosomal dissolution in Grover's disease, Hailey-Hailey's disease and Darier's disease. J Cutan Pathol 1995; 22: 488–501.

Hu CH, Michel B, Farber EM. Transient acantholytic dermatosis (Grover's disease). A skin disorder related to heat and sweating. Arch Dermatol 1985; 121: 1439–1441.

Warty Dyskeratoma

Kaddu S, Dong H, Mayer G, Kerl H, Cerroni L. Warty dyskeratoma – "follicular dyskeratoma": analysis of clinicopathologic features of a distinctive follicular neoplasm. J Am Acad Dermatol 2002; 47: 423–428.

Staphylococcal Scalded Skin Syndrome (SSSS)

Dobson CM, King CM. Adult staphylococcal scalded skin syndrome: histologic pitfalls and new diagnostic perspectives. Br J Dermatol 2003; 148: 1068–1069.

Hanakawa Y, Stanley JR. Mechanisms of blister formation by staphylococcal toxins. J Biochem 2004; 136: 747–750.

Pemphigus Foliaceus

Dasher D, Rubenstein D, Diaz LA. Pemphigus foliaceus. Curr Dir Autoimmun 2008; 10: 182–194.

Whittock NV, Bower C. Targeting of desmoglein I in inherited and acquired skin diseases. Clin Exp Dermatol 2003; 28: 410–415.

Erythema Toxicum Neonatorum

Marchini G, Ulfgren AK, Lore K, Stabi B, Berggren V, Lonne-Rahm S. Erythema toxicum neonatorum: an immunohistochemical analysis. Pediatr Dermatol 2001; 18: 177–187.

Subcorneal Pustular Dermatosis (Sneddon–Wilkinson)

Cheng S, Edmonds E, Ben-Gashir M, Yu RC. Subcorneal pustular dermatosis: 50 years on. Clin Exp Dermatol 2008; 33: 229–233.
Murphy GM, Griffiths WA. Subcorneal pustular dermatosis. Clin Exp Dermatol 1989; 14: 165–167.

Transient Neonatal Pustular Melanosis

Barr RJ, Globerman LM, Werber FA. Transient neonatal pustular melanosis. Int J Dermatol 1979; 18: 636–638.
Laude TA. Approach to dermatologic disorders in black children. Semin Dermatol 1995; 14: 15–20.

Acute Generalized Exanthematous Pustulosis (AGEP)

Beylot C, Doutre MS, Beylot-Barry M. Acute generalized exanthematous pustulosis. Semin Cutan Med Surg 1996; 15: 244–249.
Sideroff A, Halevy S, Bavinck JN, Vaillant L, Roujeau JC. Acute generalized exanthematous pustulosis (AGEP) – a clinical reaction pattern. J Cutan Pathol 2001; 28: 113–119.

Chapter 7

Granuloma Annulare

Dabski K, Winkelmann RK. Generalized granuloma annulare: histopathology and immunopathology. Systemic review of 100 cases and comparison with localized granuloma annulare. J Am Acad Dermatol 1989; 20: 28–39.

Lynch JM, Barrett TL. Collagenolytic (necrobiotic) granulomas: part 1 – the "blue" granulomas. J Cutan Pathol 2004; 31: 353–361.

Requena L, Frenandez-Figueras MT. Subcutaneous granuloma annulare. Semin Cutan Med Surg 2007; 26: 96–99.

Necrobiotic Xanthogranuloma

Lowitt MH, Dover JS. Necrobiosis lipoidica. J Am Acad Dermatol 1991; 25: 735–748.

Lynch JM, Barrett TL. Collagenolytic (necrobiotic) granulomas: part 1 – the "red" granulomas. J Cutan Pathol 2004; 31: 409–418.

Peyri J, Moreno A, Marcoval J. Necrobiosis lipoidica. Semin Cutan Med Surg 2007; 26: 87–89.

Rheumatoid Nodule

Garcia-Patos V. Rheumatoid nodule. Semin Cutan Med Surg 2007; 26: 96–99.

Ziff M. The rheumatoid nodule. Arthritis Rheum 1990; 33: 761–767.

Palisaded Neutrophilic and Granulomatous Dermatisis (Interstitial Granulomtous Dermatitis)

Chu P, Connolly MK, LeBoit PE. The histopathologic spectrum of palisaded neutrophilic and granulomatous dermatitis in patients with collagen vascular disease. Arch Dermatol 1994; 130: 1278–1283.

Verneuil L, Dompmartin A, Comoz F, Pasquier CJ, Leroy D. Interstitial granulomatous dermatitis with cutaneous cords and arthritis: a disorder associated with autoantibodies. J Am Acad Dermatol 2001; 45: 286–291.

Necrobiotic Xanthogranuloma

Fernandez-Herrera J, Pedraz J. Necrobiotic xanthogranuloma. Semin Cutan Med Surg 2007; 26: 108–113.

Mehregan DA, Winkelmann RK. Necrobiotic xanthogranuloma. Arch Dermatol 1992; 128: 94–100.

Sarcoidosis

Mangas C, Fernandez-Figueras MT, Fite E, Fernandez-Chico N, Sabat M, Fernandiz C. Clinical spectrum and histologic analysis of 32 cases of specific cutaneous sarcoidosis. J Cutan Pathol 2006; 33: 772–777.

Marchell RM, Judson MA. Chronic cutaneous lesions of sarcoidosis. Clin Dermatol 2007; 25: 295–302.

Granulomatous (Acne) Rosacea

Crawford GH, Pelle MT, James WD. Rosacea: I. Etiology, pathogenesis, and subtype classification. J Am Acad Dermatol 2004; 51: 327–341.

Cutaneous Tuberculosis

Hautmann G, Lotti T. Atypical mycobacterial infections of the skin. Dermatol Clin 1994; 12: 657–668.

MacGregor RR. Cutaneous tuberculosis. Clin Dermatol 1995; 13: 245–255.

Sehgal VN. Cutaneous tuberculosis. Dermatol Clin 1994; 12: 655–653.

Leprosy

Britton WJ, Lockwood DN. Leprosy. Lancet 2004; 363: 1209–1219.

Moschella SL. An update on the diagnosis and treatment of leprosy. J Am Acad Dermatol 2004; 51: 417–426.

Chapter 8

Leukocytoclastic Vasculitis

Carlson JA, Chen KR. Cutaneous vasculitis update: small vessel neutrophilic syndromes. Am J Dermatopathol 2006; 28: 486–506.

Chen KR, Carlson JA. Clinical approach to cutaneous vasculitis. Am J Clin Dermatol 2006; 9: 71–92.

Sams WM, Jr. Necrotizing vasculitis. J Am Acad Dermatol 1980; 3: 1–13.

Henoch–Schönlein Purpura

Lie JT. Histopathologic specificity of systemic vasculitis. Rheum Dis Clin North Am 1995; 21: 883–909.

Magro CM, Crowson AN. A clinical and histologic study of 37 cases of immunoglobulin A-associated vasculitis. Am J Dermatopathol 1999; 21: 234–240.

Erythema Elevatum Diutinum

Gibson LE, el-Azhary RA. Erythema elevatum diutinum. Clin Dermatol 2000; 18: 295–299.

Granuloma Faciale

LeBoit PE. Granuloma faciale: a diagnosis deserving of dignity. Am J Dermatopathol 2002; 24: 440–443.

Ortonne N, Weschler J, Bagot M, Grosshans E, Cribier B. Granuloma faciale: a clinicopathologic study of 66 patients. J Am Acad Dermatol 2005; 53: 1002–1009.

Cryoglobulinemia

Davis MD, Su WP. Cryoglobulinemia: recent findings in cutaneous and extracutaneous manifestations. Int J Dermatol 1996; 35: 240–248.

Goravic PD, Kassab HJ, Levo Y, Kohn R, Meltzer M, Prose P, Franklin EC. Mixed cryoglobulinemia: clinical aspects and long-term follow-up of 40 patients. Am J Med 1980; 69: 287–308.

Pityriasis Lichenoides et Varioliformis Acuta

Rogers M. Pityriasis lichenoides and lymphomatoid papulosis. Semin Dermatol 1992; 11: 73–79.

Romani J, Puig L, Frenandez-Figueras MT, de Moragas JM. Pityriasis lichenoides in children: clinicopathologic review of 22 patients. Pediatr Dermatol 1998; 15: 1–6.

Wahie S, Hiscutt E, Natarajan S, Taylor A. Pityriasis lichenoides: the differences between children and adults. Br J Dermatol 2007; 157: 941–945.

Polyarteritis Nodosa

Diaz-Perez JL, De Lagran ZM, Diaz-Ramon JL, Winkelmann RK. Cutaneous polyarteritis nodosa. Semin Cutan Med Surg 2007; 26: 77–86.

Hughes LB, Bridges SL, Jr. Polyarteritis nodosa and microscopic polyangiitis: etiologic and diagnostic considerations. Curr Rheum Rep 2002; 4: 75–82.

Jennette JC, Falk RJ, Andrassy K, Bacon PA, Churg J, Gross WL, Hagen EC, Hoffman GS, Hunter GE, Kallenberg CG. Nomenclature of systemic vasculitides: proposal of an international consensus conference. Arthritis Rheum 1994; 37: 187–192.

Superficial Thrombophlebitis

Luis Rodriguez-Peralto J, Carillo R, Rosales B, Rodriguez-Gil Y. Superficial thrombophlebitis. Semin Cutan Med Surg 2007; 26: 71–76.

Wegener's Granulomatosis

Carlson JA, Cavaliere LF, Grant-Kels JM. Cutaneous vasculitis: diagnosis and management. Clin Dermatol 2006; 24: 14–29.

Lie JT. Wegener's granulomatosis: histological documentation of common and uncommon manifestations in 216 patients. Vasa 1997; 26: 261–270.

Lynch JM. Barrett TL. Collagenolytic (necrobiotic) granulomas: part II – the 'red' granulomas. J Cutan Pathol 2004; 31: 409–418.

Allergic Granulomatosis

Lynch JM. Barrett TL. Collagenolytic (necrobiotic) granulomas: part II – the 'red' granulomas. J Cutan Pathol 2004; 31: 409–418.

Schwartz RA, Churg J. Churg–Strauss syndrome. Br J Dermatol 1992; 127: 199–204.

Chapter 9

Alopecia Areata

Eudy G, Solomon AR. The histopathology of noncicatricial alopecia. Semin Cutan Med Surg 2006; 25: 35–40.

Madani S, Shapiro J. Alopecia areata update. J Am Acad Dermatol 2000; 42: 549–566.

Wasserman D, Guzman-Sanchez DA, Scott K, McMichael A. Alopecia areata. Int J Dermatol 2007; 46: 121–131.

Secondary Syphilis

Jordaan HF, Louw M. The moth-eaten alopecia of secondary syphilis: a histopathologic study of 12 patients. Am J Dermatopathol 1995; 17: 158–162.

Follicular Mucinosis

LeBoit PE. Alopecia mucinosa, inflammatory disease or mycosis fungoides: must we choose? And are there other choices? Am J Dermatopathol 2004: 26: 167–170.

Mehregan DA, Gibson KE, Muller SA. Follicular mucinosis: histopathologic review of 33 cases. Mayo Clin Proc 1991; 66: 387–390.

Folliculitis Decalvans

Headington JT. Cicatricial alopecia. Dermatol Clin 1996; 14: 773–782.

Sperling LC. Scarring alopecia and the dermatopathologist. J Cutan Pathol 2001; 28: 333–342.

Lupus Erythematosus

McCauliffe DP. Cutaneous lupus erythematosus. Semin Cutan Med Surg 2001; 20: 14–26.

Patel P, Werth V. Cutaneous lupus erythematosus: a review. Dermatol Clin 2002; 20: 373–385.

Somani N, Bergfeld WF. Cicatricial alopecia: classification and histopathology. Dermatol Ther 2008; 21: 221–237.

Lichen Planopilaris

Mehregan DA, Van Hale HM, Muller SA. Lichen planopilaris: clinical and pathologic study of forty-five patients. J Am Acad Dermatol 1992; 27: 935–942.

Sperling LC. Scarring alopecia and the dermatopathologist. J Cutan Pathol 2001; 28: 333–342.

Tandon YK, Somani N, Cevasco NC, Bergfeld WF. A histologic review of 27 patients with lichen planopilaris. J Am Acad Dermatol 2008; 59: 91–98.

Androgenetic Alopecia

Chartier MB, Hoss DM, Grant-Kels JM. Approach to the adult female patient with diffuse nonscarring alopecia. J Am Acad Dermatol 2002; 47: 809–818.

Eudy G, Solomon AR. The histopathology of noncicatricial alopecia. Semin Cutan Med Surg 2006 25: 35–40.

Traction Alopecia (Trichotillomania)

Bergfeld WF. Alopecia: histologic changes. Adv Dermatol 1989; 301–320.

Hautmann G, Hercogova J, Lotti T. Trichotillomania. J Am Acad Dermatol 2002; 46: 807–821.

Muller SA. Trichotillomania. Dermatol Clin 1987; 5: 595–601.

Effluvium (Telogen and Anagen)

Harrison S, Sinclair R. Telogen effluvium. Clin Exp Dermatol 2002; 27: 389–395.

Headington JT. Telogen effluvium: new concepts and review. Arch Dermatol 1993; 129: 356–363.

Sperling LC. Hair and systemic disease. Dermatol Clin 2001; 19: 711–726.

Trichodystrophies

Cheng AS, Bayliss SJ. The genetics of hair shaft disorders. J Am Acad Dermatol 2008; 59: 1–22.

Chapter 10

Erythema Nodosum

Cribier B, Caille A, Heid E, Grosshans E. Erythema nodosum and associated disease: a study of 129 cases. Int J Dermatol 1998; 37: 667–672.

Mana J, Marcoval J. Erythema nodosum. Clin Dermatol 2007; 25: 288–294.

Requena L, Yus ES. Erythema nodosum. Dermatol Clin 2008; 26: 425–439.

Lupus Profundus

Fraga J, Garcia-Diaz A. Lupus erythematosus panniculitis. Dermatol Clin 2008; 26: 453–463.

Requena L, Sanchez Yus E. Panniculitis: part II. Mostly lobular panniculitis. J Am Acad Dermatol 2001; 45: 325–361.

Pancreatic Panniculitis

Dahl PR, Su WP, Cullimore KC, Dicken CH. Pancreatic panniculitis. J Am Acad Dermatol 1995; 33: 413–417.
Garcia-Romero D, Vanaclocha F. Pancreatic panniculitis. Dermatol Clin 2008; 26: 465–470.
Requena L, Sanchez Yus E. Panniculitis: part II. Mostly lobular panniculitis. J Am Acad Dermatol 2001; 45: 325–361.

α-1-Anti-trypsin Deficiency-Related Panniculitis

Requena L, Sanchez Yus E. Panniculitis: part II. Mostly lobular panniculitis. J Am Acad Dermatol 2001; 45: 325–361.
Valverde R, Rosales B, Ortiz-de Frutos FJ, Rodriguez-Peralto JL, Ortiz-Romero PL. Dermatol Clin 2008; 26: 447–451.

Weber–Christian Disease

Requena L, Sanchez Yus E. Panniculitis: part II. Mostly lobular panniculitis. J Am Acad Dermatol 2001; 45: 325–361.
White JW, Jr., Winkelmann RK. Weber–Christian panniculitis: a review of 30 cases with this diagnosis. J Am Acad Dermatol 1998; 39: 56–62.

Subcutaneous Fat Necrosis of the Newborn

Burden AD, Krafchik BR. Subcutaneous fat necrosis of the newborn: a review of 11 cases. Pediatr Dermatol 1999; 16: 384–387.
Requena L, Sanchez Yus E. Panniculitis: part II. Mostly lobular panniculitis. J Am Acad Dermatol 2001; 45: 325–361.

Factitial Panniculitis

Sammartin O, Requena C, Requena L. Factitial panniculitis. Dermatol Clin 2008; 26: 519–527.

Sclerema Neonatorum

Fretzin DF, Arias AM. Sclerema neonatorum and subcutaneous fat necrosis of the newborn. Pediatr Dermatol 1987; 4: 112–122.
Zeb A, Darmstadt GL. Sclerema neonatorum: a review of nomenclature, clinical presentation, histological features, differential diagnoses and management. J Perinatol 2008; 28: 453–460.

Erythema Induratum

Mascaro JM, Jr., Baselga E. Erythema induratum of bazin. Dermatol Clin 2008; 26: 439–445.
Requena L, Sanchez Yus E. Panniculitis. Part II. Mostly lobular panniculitis. J Am Acad Dermatol 2001; 45: 325–361.
White WL, Wieselthier JS, Hitchcock MG. Panniculitis: recent developments and observations. Semin Cutan Med Surg 1996; 15: 278–299.

Chapter 11

Lymphomatoid Papulosis

Kadin ME. Pathobiology of CD30+ cutaneous T-cell lymphomas. J Cutan Pathol 2006; 33(Suppl 1): 10–17.
Kempf W. CD30+ lymphoproliferative disorders: histopathology, differential diagnosis, new variants and simulators. J Cutan Pathol 2006; 33(Suppl 1): 58–70.
Perez A, Whittaker S. Cutaneous T-cell lymphoma. Br J Hosp Med (Lond) 2006; 67: 178–183.

Chronic Actinic Dermatosis (Actinic Reticuloid)

Menage HD, Hawk JL. The red face: chronic actinic dermatitis. Clin Dermatol 1993; 11: 297–305.
Toonstra J. Actinic reticuloid. Semin Diagn Pathol 1991; 8: 109–116.

Anti-convulsant-Induced Pseudolymphoma

Gilliam AC, Wood GS. Cutaneous lymphoid hyperplasias. Semin Cutan Med Surg 2000; 19: 133–141.
Ploysangam T, Breneman DL, Mutasim DF. Cutaneous pseudolymphomas. J Am Acad Dermatol 1988; 38: 877–895.

Gleevec-Induced Mycosis Fungoides-Like Eruption

Clark SH, Duvic M, Prieto VG. Mycosis fungoides-like reaction in a patient treated with Gleevec. J Cutan Pathol 2003; 30: 279–291.

Gianotti–Crosti Syndrome

Brandt O, Abeck D, Gianotti R, Burgdorf W. Gianotti–Crosti syndrome. J Am Acad Dermatol 2006; 54: 136–145.
Spear KL, Winkelmann RK. Gianotti–Crosti syndrome. A review of 10 cases not associated with hepatitis B. Arch Dermatol 1984; 120: 891–896.

Cutaneous Lymphoid Hyperplasia

Arai E, Shimizu M, Hirose T. A review of 55 cases of cutaneous lymphoid hyperplasia: reassessment of the histopathologic findings leading to reclassification of 4 lesions as cutaneous marginal zone lymphoma and 19 as pseudolymphomatous folliculitis. Hum Pathol 2005; 36: 505–511.

Lee MW, Lee DK, Choi JH, Koh JK. Clinicopathologic study of cutaneous pseudolymphomas. J Dermatol 2005; 32: 594–601.

Leinweber B, Colli C, Chott A, Kerl H, Cerroni L. Differential diagnosis of cutaneous infiltrates of B cells with follicular growth pattern. Am J Dermatopathol 2004; 26: 4–13.

Cutaneous Lymphadenoma

Alsadhan A, Taher M, Shokravi M. Cutaneous lymphadenoma. J Am Acad Dermatol 2003; 49: 115–116.

Okamura JM, Barr RJ. Cutaneous lymphoepithelial neoplasms. Adv Dermatol 1997; 12: 277–294.

Pardal-de-Oliveira F, Sanches A. Cutaneous lymphadenoma. Histopathology 1994; 25: 384–387.

Lymphocytic Infiltrate (of Jessner)

Mullen RH, Jacobs AH. Jessner's lymphocytic infiltrate in two girls. Arch Dermatol 1988; 124: 1091–1093.

Chapter 12

Blue Nevus

Gonzalez-Campora R, Galera-Davidson H, Vazquez-Ramirez FJ, Diaz-Cano S. Blue nevus: classical types and new related entities. A differential diagnostic review. Pathol Res Pract 1994; 190: 627–635.

Cellular Blue Nevus

Ruiter DJ, van Dijk MC, Ferrier CM. Current diagnostic problems in melanoma pathology. Semin Cutan Med Surg 2003; 22:
33–41.
Zembowicz A, Mihm MC, Jr. Dermal dendritic melanocytic
proliferations: an update. Histopathology 2004; 45: 433–451.

Nevus of Ota

Chan HH, Kono T. Nevus of Ota: clinical aspects and management. Skinmed 2003; 2: 89–96.
Grin JM, Grant-Kels JM, Grin CM, Berke A, Kels BD. Ocular
melanomas and melanocytic lesions of the eye. J Am Acad
Dermatol 1998; 38: 716–730.
Zembowicz A, Mihm MC, Jr. Dermal dendritic melanocytic
proliferations: an update. Histopathology 2004; 45: 433–451.

Nevus of Ito

De Giotgi V, Sestini S, Massi D, Lotti T. Melanocytic aggrega-
tion in the skin: diagnostic clues from lentigines to melanoma.
Dermatol Clin 2007; 25: 303–320.
Zembowicz A, Mihm MC, Jr. Dermal dendritic melanocytic
proliferations: an update. Histopathology 2004; 45: 433–451.

Mongolian Spot

Zembowicz A, Mihm MC, Jr. Dermal dendritic melanocytic
proliferations: an update. Histopathology 2004; 45: 433–451.

Chlorpromazine Hyperpigmentation

Hashimoto K, Joselow SA, Tye MJ. Imipramine hyperpigmentation: a slate-gray discoloration caused by long-term

imipramine administration. J Am Acad Dermatol 1991; 25: 357–361.

Zelickson AS. Skin pigmentation and chlorpromazine. JAMA 1965: 194: 670–672.

Regression

Barnhill RL. Pathology and prognostic factors. Curr Opin Oncol 1993; 5: 364–376.

Byers HR, Bhawan J. Pathologic parameters in the diagnosis and prognosis of primary cutaneous melanoma. Hematol Oncol North Am 1998; 12: 717–735.

Hussein MR. Tumour-infiltrating lymphocytes and melanoma tumorigenesis: an insight. Br J Dermatol 2005; 153: 18–21.

Murphy GF, Mihm MC, Jr. Histologic reporting of malignant melanoma. Monogr Pathol 1988; 30: 79–93.

Woods GM, Malley RC, Muller HK. The skin immune system and the challenge of tumour immunosurveillance. Eur J Dermatol 2005; 15: 63–69.

Argyria

Granstein RD, Sober AJ. Drug- and heavy metal-induced hyper-pigmentation. J Am Acad Dermatol 1981; 5: 1–18.

Chrysiasis

Granstein RD, Sober AJ. Drug- and heavy metal-induced hyper-pigmentation. J Am Acad Dermatol 1981; 5: 1–18.

Hemochromatosis

Chevrant-Breton J, Simon M, Bourel M, Ferrand B. Cutaneous manifestations of idiopathic hemochromatosis. Study of 100 cases. Arch Dermatol 1977; 113: 161–165.

Minocycline Hyperpigmentation

Bohm M, Schmidt PF, Lodding B, Uphoff H, Westermann G, Luger TA, Bonsmann G, Metze D. Cutaneous hyperpigmentation induced by doxycycline: histochemical and ultrastructural examination, laser microprobe mass analysis and cathodoluminescence. Am J Dermatopathol 2002; 24: 345–350.

Bowen AR, MacCalmont TH. The histopathology of subcutaneous minocycline pigmentation. J Am Acad Dermatol 2007; 57: 836–839.

Mouton RW, Jordaan HF, Schneider JW. A new type of minocycline-induced cutaneous hyperpigmentation. Clin Exp Dermatol 2004; 29: 8–14.

Ochronosis

Kramer KE Lopez A, Stefanato CM, Phillips TJ. Exogenous ochronosis. J Am Acad Dermatol 2000; 42: 869–871.

Touart DM, Sau P. Cutaneous deposition diseases. Part II. J Am Acad Dermatol 1998; 39: 527–544.

Amiodarone Pigmentation

Dootson G, Byatt G. Amiodarone-induced vasculitis and a review of the cutaneous side-effects of amiodarone. Clin Exp Dermatol 1994; 19: 422–424.

Fitzpatrick JE. New histopathologic findings in drug eruptions. Dermatol Clin 1992; 10: 19–36.

Index